Ironmom

TRAINING & RACING IN A FAMILY OF SEVEN

METTE HARRISON

Ironmom

TRAINING & RACING IN A FAMILY OF SEVEN

Published by Familius LLC, www.familius.com

Familius books are available at special discounts for bulk purchases for sales promotions, family or corporate use. Special editions, including personalized covers, excerpts of exist-ing books, or books with corporate logos, can be created in large quantities for special needs. For more information, contact Premium Sales at 559-876-2170 or email special-markets@familius.com

Library of Congress Catalog-in-Publication Data

2013933819

pISBN: 978-1-938301-36-0
eISBN: 978-1-938301-35-3

Printed in the United States of America

Edited by Michele Robbins
Cover design by David Miles
Book design by Maggie Wickes

10 9 8 7 6 5 4 3 2 1

First Edition

TABLE OF CONTENTS

INTRODUCTION

People who know me now imagine that I have always been athletic, always driven, always interested in racing. This isn't true. When I was a child, my only interest in athletics was in having fun. I enjoyed walking around our big yard in central New Jersey. I enjoyed chasing after our dog and the chickens on the big two-acre lot that my parents had made into a farm. I remember our pony Romeo and how much I loved to ride him.

But at school, it was all different. There, I hated running the mile in PE classes and would do anything I could to avoid the continual sense that I was overweight, slow, and that my body was somehow just made wrong because I was in so much pain. I was convinced that nothing could ever change, that I was always going to be the kid no one wanted on any recess kickball team.

The summer when I was fifteen, I have a distinct memory of going on a rafting trip down the Colorado River with a group of neighbors and a handful of adults who were our supervisors. It rained almost the entire time, a miserable and unusual week in a Utah summer. But on Thursday afternoon, there was a beautiful burst of sunshine. We stopped for lunch on shore and let our clothes dry out for a bit. Then, after the food had settled, we kids started to chase the adults in an impromptu game. We were trying to throw them into the river (to get wet again).

I remember how much fun I had running that afternoon. I remember the sun shining down on me and how glorious it felt. I remember the feeling of my bare feet in the sand as I ran. I wasn't trying to get a gym teacher to give me a decent grade. I didn't care about my time or how my body looked jiggling along the track. I just wanted to be part of a team of kids who were ganging up on the adults and throwing them in the river. And I loved it! I loved the sensation of running with a group, with a purpose. I loved how I felt in my own body; I wasn't being judged. I loved pushing myself as hard as I wanted to push.

Sadly, once we got back in the rafts and headed home, I did not feel that sense of pure pleasure in running for a long time again, or in anything else athletic, really. I worked hard at swim team, but without many results. Anxiety got in my way, that sense of being judged and being found wanting that I think many of us feel, in so many parts of our lives. I grew up and my body started to creak. I went to doctors who told me to do less and less. I stopped walking and started to dread the stairs. I gained weight with each baby, and it did not come back off.

And then one day, I fought back against all that. I found a doctor who was interested in helping me get back to what I used to do, who I used to be—if only for that one afternoon. I wanted to be again the person who was comfortable in her body and who loved to move. So I signed up for a marathon where it wasn't about finishing in a certain time. There was no prize to be won as far as I could see. It was just about me and the distance, me doing something that I had thought so impossible I had never even considered putting it on a list of goals. I finished that race, and then I signed up for others. I completed them, and then I did more than complete them. I triumphed over them.

There are still days when it rains in the raft, when I just huddle under a tarp and wish that the day was over. But there are more and more days in my life when I get out and find sunshine, either outside or in my own exercise room. I chase down my own demons or I simply let myself go back to that one moment as a teenager when I felt good about my body, when I pushed myself because I wanted to push myself.

At my most recent race, Race in Las Vegas April 20, 2013, I forgot my watch. I did the entire race without any idea of what my time was. It wasn't my best race. I ended up with a flat tire and that was frustrating. But not having a watch made it so that I really had no idea how much time I was losing. And that was a great thing. Instead of the race being about a time, it was once again about me and my body, me facing a challenge. A challenge that I choose for myself, and that only I judged the results of.

The best races are a chance for me to be once again the teenage girl who realized that running didn't always have to be about not being good enough. The best races aren't about feeling fat or awkward or in the wrong shoes because I couldn't afford better ones. They are about me doing what I want to do, making myself do something that would have seemed impossible if anyone else had asked me to do it. But since I am doing it for me, I can't rebel and most importantly of all, I can't fail. I can only find out who I am, and that is the person who always turns out to be surprised at what she can do.

In triathlon, I have also learned things about other people that I will never forget. People who stop and help other racers when they don't have to, simply because they like to help. People who go on with incredible injuries to finish races simply because they won't give up. People who cheer me on after I have passed them because they feel the spirit of togetherness in a race.

Triathlon is one of the kindest communities in the world. I have never been to a race where people did not want to help each other out in some way. A flat by the side of the road elicits offers of a tube or air. People who get injured and can't race come and volunteer at aid stations or just cheer along the way. And when the last person crosses the finish line, whether bleeding, or in his seventies, or sixty pounds overweight, we all cheer because we are all racing the same race, against ourselves, not each other.

Come join my community. Come read about my adventure to come to where I am today. It's not an endeavor for the faint of heart, but it is for anyone who is willing to give back one hundred percent. I have found happiness, peace, and not a small part of my best self here—in the water, on the bike, out running hills. That's why I wrote this book. Whenever I talked about it, people would shake their heads and tell me that I sounded passionate, that I almost made them believe they could do it. And you can do it! Any of you can!

CHAPTER 1

WHY TRI?

I signed up for Ironman Coeur d'Alene on September 5, 2005, one week after I delivered my sixth child, Mary Mercy—stillborn. I had tried a triathlon briefly in 2004, and had kept in shape during the pregnancy, mostly by swimming. I had intended to do an Ironman one day in a sort of mystical far off future, after this last baby was born. But I discovered I desperately needed to do it as part of my recovery from grief. Maybe this makes no sense, adding something else to an already busy life with five other children and grief to deal with as well, but I needed focus and purpose—and training for an Ironman twenty or more hours a week certainly gives you that.

Mary Mercy

My due date was August 20 and Mercy was still not here. My second child, Sage, had been a week overdue and Faith, my fourth child, had been eight days overdue. Those last days when you are overdue, when friends and family call and ask if there is good news yet, when people stop you in the street and ask when is that baby coming—each day is like a month of the torture of the previous pregnancy. I admit, I hate being pregnant. I suffer pre-partum depression and am one of those people who is instantly better as soon as I give birth. Literally, moments after the cord is cut, I will be ready to get up and start walking around, being in my own body again. This is one of the reasons that I have delivered most of my kids at home with the help of a lay midwife, rather than in a hospital.

I feel an enormous rush of energy after birth and the only thing that keeps me going during those last months of pregnancy is the knowledge that I will get a baby out of this. There is nothing I love more than a newborn. I am in heaven with a newborn. I don't really even feel a need for help with meals or caring for my family...once the baby is here. I am myself again. Even getting three to four hours of sleep a night does not faze me. I am always eager to get home and get back to my real life with my other kids. With several babies, I have had to check out of the hospital AMA (Against Medical Advice) because doctors didn't want to release me two hours after delivery.

For Mercy, I had planned a home birth as well. I was working with a new midwife whom I trusted. She had a backup doctor on call if there were any problems during the delivery. She also had an ultrasound machine, and although she wasn't professionally trained to read ultrasounds, things looked fine with the baby, whom we had found out was a girl at about twenty weeks. We chose the name Mary Mercy to go with our family tradition. The children have a first name that is after a family member and a second name that is a quality we admire. The girls have all ended up going by their middle names. Our children are Shannon Hope (1994), Hannah Sage (1995), Samuel Worthy (1997), Emily Faith (1999), Zachary Mark (2002), and Mary Mercy (2005) to be called Mercy.

We started calling the baby "Mercy" as soon as we knew she was a girl at twenty weeks. Hope, my oldest, was very much in love with her little sister. She would sing to Mercy and talk to her inside my stomach and play little in utero kicking games. Hope was so excited with the idea of having a new little person to play with and take care of. Hope is very nurturing and I knew she would be an amazing big sister.

The morning of August 29, I woke up knowing immediately that something was wrong. Ironically, I had slept through the night, which a heavily pregnant woman never does. The baby simply kicks too much and you have to move too many times. I realized when I woke that the baby had not kicked all night. I tried to eat some food to get the baby to move, but nothing happened. Sick at heart, I woke Matt up and told him that the baby hadn't been moving. Normally, Matt is very logical and does not panic easily. For about ten seconds, he was ready to dismiss my concerns. Then he came over, felt my belly, and could feel that it wasn't right. He called the midwife, who assured us over the phone that everything would be fine. But, as soon as she arrived, she tried to find the baby's heartbeat and couldn't. Matt knew that the baby was gone, but I held to the hope that the Doppler machine was wrong and that we would get to the hospital and find everything was OK.

We left the children with a neighbor to help them get to school. We did not tell them anything was wrong. As soon as the hospital did an ultrasound, they changed us from delivery status to still-born status with a sign on the door to make sure that people didn't come in and do insensitive things like talk to us about nursing the baby after birth. Then Matt made a series of painful phone calls to people who had been expecting good news. Matt's parents had been through a stillbirth years before, though much earlier on in the pregnancy. They immediately began to drive to the hospital with Matt's brother, Ben. Matt called my parents, who were far away in Nauvoo, Illinois.

Then we got visitors who had been through stillbirths as well and helped talk us through it. They explained our options in terms of cremation or burial, talked to us about taking photos with the baby and perhaps some hand molds to remember her. I felt almost no pain as I was put on Pitocin, a drug that mimics natural hormones to produce labor. For the next two hours I was in labor with no epidural or painkillers. Matt's parents and brother had arrived and we spent that time talking about triathlons and my hopes for the future. Ben and his wife Amanda had been training to do some small triathlons and he asked me for advice about nutrition, spacing of races, and anything else he could think of. I was conscious of the fact that this was probably a strange conversation to be having under the circumstances, but Ben explained to me later he figured this was just distraction, like talking to a little kid with a broken arm about the next baseball game. It worked. For a little while, I didn't think about how horrible it was to have lost a baby and to have to go through labor anyway. I didn't think about what I would tell my children or how my life would change.

Finally, I was ready to deliver and Matt's parents and brother excused themselves. The baby was born and our children came to the hospital. Matt explained what had happened to little Mercy. They were all teary. Faith was a little afraid of the baby. Zach simply said, "When she is alive again, we will play with her." Hope and Sage felt cheated after all the waiting for the baby. We took a few photos and then our children went home with Matt's parents. We drove home later, after the epidural had worn off and I could stand up again. To drive home without a baby after an intense labor and delivery was agony. That night was difficult, as we had to plan a funeral as well as deal with the same physical healing as any mother who has gone through a delivery. Pain, bleeding, cramps. In the morning, for the first time in a long time, I did no workout.

On the third day, I wrote in my workout journal that I went out power walking. The fourth day, I was starting to run a little here and there. Yes, I know this is exactly NOT what you are supposed to do. One of the women in my neighborhood who is a labor and delivery nurse and also a runner saw me out one of those early mornings and gave me a talking to, "You don't want to end up in the hospital with a hemorrhage on top of everything else." But honestly, I was not in a state of mind to care about that. I only wanted to get out running, to feel the rush of adrenaline in my system again, and to feel like I had something in my life other than pain and grief. I wanted to be normal again; I wanted to push out the emotional pain any way I could.

From a Grieving Heart to a Training Heart

Once I had signed up for the Ironman and was officially cleared to train by my doctor, I began head on. I loved the physical charge of the adrenaline rush. It helped me feel good for hours afterward. Every day I could check off another step on my list towards achieving a goal that was within my control. I had failed as an athlete in high school, but I went back to it as an adult and had felt an enormous sense of redemption in being able to conquer something that most adults have given up on. Losing Mercy left me feeling crushed by fate. I wanted to be in control of my own life again. And I wanted to triumph over something.

I spent weeks getting up at 5:00 in the morning, then 4:00, then 3:00. I had five children and a career as a writer that I had to juggle with my training. My goal was to finish by 8:00 a.m. so that we could have family scripture time and breakfast together before they all went off to school. I wanted to keep my children from making sacrifices for me, so I tried to insulate them from the terrible grief that I felt more deeply than they did. But of course, that did not happen. They watched me struggle after workouts that burned up my legs, my brain, and my heart. They lived without my direction through Saturday chores when I was out on the bike. However, they reaped the benefits of my eating chocolate cake almost every day in attempt to keep up the calories. I think they miss that part.

Five weeks before the race, I drove up to Coeur D'Alene so that I could bike the actual course and see the hills I would have to conquer. It was pouring rain, which seems pretty normal in a place that is on the border of Oregon and Washington.

Finally, after seven months of training, Matt took off work, we loaded the five kids and my gear in the car, and we headed off for a sort of family vacation.

Matt's younger sister, her husband, and her two children happened to live in Coeur D'Alene and we would be staying with them. The only difficulty for me there was that she had a baby girl who had been due within days of Mercy. Her name was Lily, and she had come to the funeral. It had been good to hear a baby there when I couldn't have my own, but there were also times when seeing her reminded me of my loss. It wasn't her fault or her mother's, and I knew that. In fact, Emily's husband Michael had given us an enormously generous gift of a handmade cedar chest with Mary Mercy carved on the front of it. To this day we keep all of the memorabilia we gathered from her birth: photos, flowers, cards, and things we did not want to give away—things that had been meant to be hers.

We all went out on the lake the day before the race. The kids had a grand time while I tried to stay down and keep my legs rested. It is a beautiful area, so green and thickly wooded. The water was gorgeous and blue; the sky was perfectly clear. We walked around the race finish line where there were vendors set up selling last minute items. I tried out my wetsuit in the cold water and thought about how lucky I was to have the equipment, the family support, and the physical health to do this.

Ironmom

I went to sleep fairly easily the night before the race, which was a good thing. I had been suffering from grief-induced insomnia for months. My only solution was to get up at midnight when I couldn't sleep and get on the treadmill. Sometimes I would run twelve or fourteen miles before I decided I was tired enough to collapse into bed.

I woke up at 5:00 in the morning of the Ironman in early June 2006. Matt drove me to the beach to start the swim in a beautiful, but quite cold (about sixty degrees) lake. I put on my Body Glide and wetsuit, got body marked with my official race number, put last minutes items in my bags, and checked my bike tires one last time. Then I put on my sunscreen. The day was already hot and was predicted to be a record breaker.

I stood on the shore of the beach and looked out at the buoys that marked the course. There would be two loops in the swim. In between each loop, we would have to get out, run along the beach, and prove by running over a timer that we had done the first loop. The announcer told us there were over four thousand volunteers there, to help two thousand athletes finish. There was an incredible spirit of energy with all of the athletes standing together and the crowds behind us of family, friends, news people, and volunteers cheering for us. We counted down from ten all together, and the race began.

The swim start was nerve wracking as two thousand athletes (men and women) started into the water at the same time. It was impossible not to get knocked in the face, stomach, or crotch many, many times. And yet, they were all there, doing the same thing, struggling through the same water, fighting to get the same air. Around the buoys we went. In the photograph I was given afterwards, we looked like a long snake with a thin head and a thin tail, but with most of us in the middle somewhere thrashing through. I climbed out of the water roughly in the middle, placing

770th. Matt had stayed to watch the swim and to see me get out of the water. He called out my name, waved to me, and then headed back home to get the kids dressed and ready for church. He would be coming in and out with kids to cheer me along my way.

I finished the 2.4 mile swim in about 1:10 (exactly 35 minutes per loop) then ran into the huge transition area. There were a dozen people waiting to help me out of my wetsuit. All I had to do was sit down and they pulled it off. Then another volunteer got my bag for me, dumped it out and asked if I needed help putting anything on. Another volunteer waited with sunscreen to apply—a top priority for me in the unusual ninety-five degree heat that was expected that day. It had been raining when I previewed the course, and the day before they had still been predicting seventy degree weather. They were wrong. I took a long drink of Gatorade from another volunteer and hit the toilets.

Then I was on my bike, heading out for the first loop. I saw a couple of athletes I knew from Utah and greeted them briefly as I went. Every one of us had our names on our backs, so we could call out and encourage each other. I had fun listening to people try to pronounce my name, and end up just cheering me by number— 2139. I was watching my heart rate carefully. Though there were a lot of hills on this course, my coach had told me that I had to keep my heart rate under 150 at all times, and under 142 as an average on both the run and the bike. I had done well in training keeping my heart rate at 142 or lower on the bike, but had almost never managed to keep my heart rate that low while running for more than thirty minutes. But, I was going to try.

Every ten miles on the bike course there were about sixty volunteers waiting—apparently their sole purpose in life being to hand out ice cold bottles of Gatorade or water, sports gels, power bars, or bananas. They would stand in a long line, with arms outstretched, and if you shouted what you wanted, they would approach to make sure you could grab what you needed without slowing down. If you missed, there was another person further down. Occasionally, there were collisions between cyclists and sometimes between cyclists and volunteers, but considering how many chances for mishap there were, it was amazing there weren't more.

As I biked I saw a racer off her bike on the side of the road in one of the tricky sections of the course. This really shook me up. In Coeur D'Alene in 2006, there was a long section of sharply steep hills and equally sharply downhill sections. The uphill sections were brutal and I saw a lot of people walking up them, particularly the second loop of the course. It was sensible, considering how much energy you might use up on an uphill that you might not recover. Going too fast early in the race costs you twice as many minutes (at least) as you think it is saving you.

But it was the downhill that was worse. If you are going absolutely straight, you can let your bike go fast. And yes, if you watch the Tour de France you will see cyclists going seventy miles an hour on those fast switchbacks. That is insane in my opinion, and people do die at those speeds with only a helmet on. I have always had the strategy of safety first on a bike and I annoyed those cyclists behind me who wanted to go faster but were forced by the rules of triathlon not to draft and to wait to pass me. I do not take chances on sharp turns. I slow way down.

The racer I saw on the side of the road had taken one chance too many. She was bleeding and broken and was not getting up. There was, thankfully, already a team of people around her waiting for an ambulance. We saw in the paper the next day that she had survived, but was in pretty bad shape, the one really serious casualty of the day. Ironman is not for wimps, and it's not for the reckless either.

By the end of the final loop of the bike, I was really feeling the heat and, I suspect, I was rather dehydrated. I had not been used to training in high temperatures this early in the season, and I had also not anticipated a rather long section without aid at the end of the loop. I saw Matt and the kids near the end both times, though I was a little late on the second loop. I had expected to finish each loop in 3 hours, but had slowed to 3:20 on the second time around. Matt was still there though, cheering me ahead with the words that I had preapproved. I warned him in advance that the worst thing for me would be to hear him shouting at me to go faster. An Ironman race is so long that your worst enemy is going too fast early on. You want to keep going at a steady pace that you can easily maintain, but I am very competitive and I worried that if he shouted at me to go faster, I would forget my goals. I told him instead that he and the kids should shout things like, "Keep hydrated," "Hold your pace," and, "Slow and steady." They did that very well.

My official bike time was 6:25. As soon as I got off my bike, it was taken by a volunteer and brought back to its proper place along the bike racks. Meanwhile I was ushered forward to a cool tent where a wonderful woman put an ice cold towel on my neck and on my chest. She brought me a cup of Gatorade to hydrate and a cup of ice to put down my bra. It sounds terrible, but if you have ever been truly overheated or in a long race, you will understand how wonderful it actually feels to be cooled off from as close to the core of your body as you can get. I put ice water on my head and put ice in my hat as well. Then the woman helped me off with my bike shoes and socks, and put on my run shoes and socks. Another volunteer reapplied sunscreen to my back. I sat quietly for a moment, trying to collect myself.

The cold-towel woman sat down next to me and told me that I was her hero. She couldn't believe I had done so well, that I had come so far, and she told me she knew I would finish. She was my hero too.

I got out on the run, struggled, and realized quickly that my goal pace of ten minutes per mile and my goal run time of 4:30 was going to be impossible. Even finishing seemed out of reach as my heart rate skyrocketed into the 170s. To get my heart rate under the recommended 150 beats per minute I had to stop and walk after three miles of running. It took about two miles for it to drop into the 120s. At that point I felt good enough that I could consider running again. But I couldn't run for long, only about five minutes, before my heart rate went up again. This was partly because of the heat and partly because I simply wasn't a good enough runner to be able to keep my heart rate low after almost ten hours of exercise.

Running has always been the weakest of the three disciplines of triathlon for me, and it doesn't help that it comes last when I am utterly exhausted. Sometimes people ask me why they would do the swim first in triathlon when temperatures are hottest at the end. It would make more sense in some ways to put the swim in the middle or whenever it will be hottest. But the reality is that when you are doing an ultra-distance event like this, safety has to be the first concern. You want people in the water when they are at their strongest, because you don't want anyone drowning. You want people on the bike for the second section because if you get too tired, the risks of falling off your bike at speed are still pretty high. The run is the least dangerous of the three sports. All that happens to you if you collapse while running is that you fall to the ground. You can survive that. I've seen it happen plenty of times.

As I headed up the first hill of the course, I saw the leading professional women cross my path. They were almost done, and they had bikes in front of them with signs to tell who they were. I was a good twenty miles behind all of them. The twenty or so professional triathletes started thirty minutes earlier than the rest of the two thousand amateur athletes. Still, I was far behind the best amateurs, who are nearly as good as the pros. Nonetheless, professionals and amateurs, experienced and inexperienced, we were all on the same course. This has long been one of the unique aspects of an Ironman race. Where else do you see the profession-als running the same course at the same time as the amateurs? It leads to a real sense of solidarity and healthy competition.

There were people standing by the side of the road near their houses asking if racers wanted to be pelted with water from a hose. Almost all of us did. There were aid stations every mile, which was crucial for me. Instead of thinking about the whole twenty-six miles, you could think about one mile at a time. Just get to the aid station, and you'll be fine, I tell myself. While I was walking, I would pass people who would encourage me to run, but there were lots of times when I just couldn't run. I was doing the best I could. I finished the first loop of the run, the second half of which was downhill, and I was still struggling mightily.

I began to tell myself that all I had to do was walk, that I'd finish if I walked, and if I felt better later, I could run. I went through twenty miles of the marathon, running when I could, walking the rest. It was an impressive lesson in the absolute limits of my body's functions. I simply felt like I was going to throw up and pass out if my heart rate hit 170. When I let it drop again, I felt more optimistic about the prospect of finishing the course.

By the end of the first loop of the run, I had seen a lot of people pass me, and a lot of grown men puking their guts out by the side of the road and then proceeding to a walk that was somehow even slower than mine. I also saw one man being escorted away from the water's edge by two security guards. There were plenty of people in the water swimming, so I couldn't figure out what he'd done wrong until I saw he had a race number on. As he passed by me, I heard him muttering, "I have to get in the water, I have to do the Ironman." He'd already finished the swim and bike, but he didn't remember anymore. The security guard next to him said, "Sir, you're confused because of severe dehydration. We have to get you to a medical tent immediately." He was only one of the unlucky ones. Every Ironman has a certain number of DNF's (Did Not Finisher's). The hotter it is, and the worse the wind, the higher the number. It was a lot hotter (ninety-five degrees Fahrenheit) in Coeur D'Alene that year than any of us had expected or trained for.

It was starting to get dark by the time I hit mile twenty-three. Cooler temperatures meant that I felt a lot better and my heart rate no longer seemed to be spiking so easily. I made a goal to finish the last three miles of the race running all the way. I passed probably 150 people, because many athletes had not left enough energy for the end of the race. It is so hard to pace yourself properly for a race that long. For most races, a 5k or a 10k, you have a chance to do the full distance in training. Even in a marathon, you do close to the full distance. Some runners do twenty miles, some twenty-three as their longest long runs. Others do a full twenty-six miles or more if they are very serious or are confident in their abilities and their luck in not getting injured. But in an Ironman, where many people have a final time of more than fifteen hours, it's just impossible to do a training day that is near that long. The strategy many people use is to do a bike on Saturday that is close to 112 miles, and then on Sunday do a long run up to twenty miles, back to back. I had never been able to do this because I didn't want to train on Sundays. So, I did a long run on Wednesday and a long bike on Saturday. Perhaps, in retrospect, that hadn't been the best plan.

At last, I could see the finish line. I ran through, heard my name called (mispronounced) and was declared an "Ironman." My finish time was 13:06. I finished the marathon in 5:15. I missed my goal, but finished faster than many. I finished in 853rd place. I walked through the finishing chute in agony, though I had been running moments before. I felt certain that I would never do this again, ever. I was violently nauseated, nearly every muscle torn and protesting. I told Matt I thought I needed to go to the hospital, because this couldn't possibly be the way it was supposed to feel. But more than the physical pain was the painful disappointment with my time and my weaknesses. I focused on the failed goal, not the accomplishment—not able to appreciate what I had done, because it was less than perfect.

It reminded me of that other day, when I was also imperfect, and my body had not been able to keep the placenta that kept Mercy alive functioning. Matt said that he thought the Ironman preparation was like a pregnancy in many ways—all those months of preparation leading to an unknown that did not turn out as I had hoped. But, it was also a reminder that even in the very darkest moments of life, total strangers can help you along, and maybe make you smile a little. That was true of both the Ironman and Mercy's stillbirth—total strangers who came to my rescue simply because I needed it. I had lived through a marathon of grief and then a through a triple marathon of Ironman.

One of the best aid stations on the run had a group of a dozen grandmotherly ladies dressed in clown wigs and muumuus, waving fuzzy sticks around and dancing wildly to loud music. Crazy stuff, but if it distracts you for just one minute, they've done their job. I know that there are bad things that happen everywhere, but I have seen such overwhelming goodness from people I did not know. The woman who helped ice me down before I started the run. The woman who sat and explained to me what a stillborn baby would look like, so that I would be prepared to face the black fingernails and gray skin. The volunteers who handed me Gatorade, pretzels, and chicken broth when I needed it. The notes, cards, gifts, flowers, and food I received from people I barely knew. My sister, who took over the burden of calling the whole family for me. The gift of the cedar chest. The gift of a photo-shopped image of Mercy, worked on all night by one of Matt's old work friends so that we could have it at the funeral. A hundred tiny gifts.

My kids called me "Ironmom" after I was finished. We went home, and I was determined that we were going to be a family— that what I had suffered would not make me less of a mom than I had been before. I thought I was done with Ironman, though I knew I would do more triathlons. I was wrong. Ironman and triathlon were both more powerful draws than I had realized, and I have needed again and again the distraction and the sense of purpose that training and racing provide. I have also enjoyed the sense of triumph and accomplishment, and have begun to share that with my children.

Tips for Getting Started

Make a Reasonable Commitment.

How much time are you going to devote to working out? Write it down in minutes. How many days a week are you going to do this? If you are moving from being a couch potato, it is not reasonable to expect you will be able to do an hour of working out a day. Even walking or easy biking should be approached gently. ten minutes the first day is plenty. Fifteen minutes the next day. Then ten minutes again. Gradually go up, not increasing your speed until you have been doing an hour of exercise per day for at least a month. Then you can try to get faster, but only if you keep your exercise level at an hour and do not increase it. Make sure you get an OK from your doctor so you know if you have any restrictions. Most doctors will be happy to encourage you because they know that exercise dramatically improves a patient's health.

Look for Beginner's Classes at Your Local Gym

Ask someone at the desk for a recommendation. You don't want to do BodyPump to begin with and many spin classes are for more advanced people, so if you are beginning find the beginner's class. If you are great at cycling already, look for help in the other two sports. You can sometimes find a master's swim team for beginners where you will get tips on improving your swimming. There are also great yoga classes and I love Pilates for beginners.

Running is largely solitary, but you can occasionally find runner's groups online in your area. More advanced groups meet at a track regularly to encourage healthy competition. But just finding someone who runs at your pace and is willing to meet at a regular, set time, can be enormously helpful to keep you in the habit. Ask in your neighborhood or watch other runners you see out on the street while driving or running to see if they are the right pace. Don't do all of your workouts with others, because you need to make sure you are doing what you need to do, but you can do at least half of them in a group.

Find a Trainer to Help You Get Started.

A trainer is a great person to help you figure out how to use the weight equipment at the gym and what sorts of exercises you should be doing. If you can't afford a trainer, maybe you can find a friend who would be willing to let you shadow him/her for a few weeks at the gym. Even better, find someone who is just a little better than you are and who would be willing to be your workout buddy. Then you will have someone to help show you the way and make it more fun to workout. Weightlifting is really important, especially as we age, to counteract the tendency to lose muscle mass. Don't skip on this part of your training plan. Try to get in two weight training workouts a week. Start slowly and try to avoid making yourself really sore the next day.

Reward Yourself

You can reward yourself with money on a regular basis, like five dollars for each hour of working out to spend on new clothes. Or, if you workout at home in front of the TV, reward yourself with movies and TV shows you want to see. If you need food rewards, make them small and moderately healthy. Sometimes we think we deserve a piece of cheesecake after a long workout, but it's rare that you will be burning the one thousand calories most cheese-cake slices have. Think of a yummy fresh mango or berry shake instead.

Be Accountable.

Make an achievable goal and keep track of your progress toward the goal. There are online communities set up to help you do this, some free, some not. But I am sometimes uncomfortable letting other people see my goals, even if I'm doing well. So I just keep an inexpensive, lined paper notebook at my desk and write down a week's worth of workouts on every page. I write down how long I worked out, at what pace or how many calories I burned, and then I sometimes write notes about how I felt like "crappy," "sick," or "great!" I like being able to look back sometimes and see how far I've come, but I doubt anyone else would be able to figure out what my notebooks means. That's fine. It's not for them. It's for me and I know what it means.

Give Yourself a Budget

You will need to spend some money to make it interesting and safe to keep working out. You will probably need to purchase a gym membership. Even if you are planning to walk (which is just fine for my mother and for lots of people), you will want a place you can walk during the winter. Maybe you can go to the local mall. You can do it for a low cost, but you will probably still need some good shoes. If you have higher aspirations for racing, make sure that you budget the cost for the entry fees, travel, and food. At the beginning of every year, I try to set a budget for race fees and remember which ones really matter to me. It's easy to get sucked into every race that comes along, but it isn't good for your training to race more than about once a month. We also try to stick to a budget for repairs on bikes and racing food as well as an entertainment budget for going out to eat the night before a race or sometimes for lunch after a race. Don't bankrupt yourself. If all you can afford is an exercise ball and a yoga mat for your weight training, that's fine. There's a lot you can do with those simple tools. Make goals that work with the resources you have.

Get the Proper Gear

Once you have set a budget, you can go shopping. Don't spend your entire budget on the first shopping trip. You will discover you need things along the way. But don't nickel and dime yourself, either. Good running shoes cost money. Don't buy them at Payless or Walmart. Don't try to get by with a swimsuit that doesn't fit you anymore. Don't wear goggles that leak. You will hate your workouts if you do not have adequate gear, and then you will stop doing them.

Make Realistic Goals

If you want to do a race, make sure that you set it far enough out that you can train for it. A shorter race takes less time to train for, obviously. And if something happens or you get injured, have a back-up plan for another race that you could do as an alternative at a later date. Make goals that are completely dependent on you and your persistence, not on other people or on wildly optimistic plans of the future. For example, a goal of finishing a race is reasonable. A goal of winning a race is not reasonable because you don't know who else will be at the race. You can't determine what other people will do—only what you will do. I often set a best-case scenario goal, a medium goal where things go well but not perfectly, and then a backup goal if everything goes badly but I still want to be proud of myself for trying.

Don't Give Up

If you don't see the results you want to see, don't just assume that the laws of the universe work for everyone else and not you. That's just silly. We know the principles for improving fitness and weight. Stick with them, even when it seems like you're not seeing results. If you need to get a different scale to help you see that even if you're not losing weight, you're changing your body composition, put it into the budget. These scales are surprisingly accurate at showing changes. If you are working out, your fat percent will go down even when your weight doesn't. And if you want to lose weight, then make sure that you are accurately reporting your daily calorie intake and expenditure.

Keep People around You Who Are Cheering for You to Succeed.

This is true in all areas of life, not just in triathlon training. I am not someone who likes to train with other people. I like solitary contemplation, but everyone needs people who are cheering. If you have someone in your life whose voice is in your mind when you are at your lowest and that voice tells you to quit, that is someone you need out of your life—or you need them to change. By the same token, spend more time with people who encourage you, whose voices you hear when you are at your lowest, telling you to keep going, that they believe in you. If you have people in your life who are accidentally sabotaging you, feel free to tell them honestly and kindly that you need something else. Give them a script with appropriate comments to make, like I did with Matt and the kids on the Ironman. When they do what you need, you will know that they are on your team.

CHAPTER 2

I NEVER CLEAN OUT MY REFRIGERATOR, AND OTHER CONFESSIONS OF A TRIATHLETE

Some people wonder how I take care of five kids, write fiction novels, play piano, knit, quilt, and train for ten or fifteen triathlons a year. Well, it's pretty simple. I skip a lot of stuff that other people do every day. There's a simple rule that if you want to add something into your life, you have to give up something. I'm not super woman, not really. I just have priorities and I am fierce about protecting them.

Everyone has the same twenty-four hours in each day. If you use eight of those to sleep and two to eat and bathe, that leaves you fourteen hours. Decide what you want to do with them. If you truly have nothing you are willing to give up, and nothing from which you are willing to cut off time, you are not going to be able to exercise. You can't make time. Don't expect the impossible from yourself or from the universe. You will only be disappointed and frustrated. The truth is that almost everyone can find time to do some exercise if they are willing to examine their schedule and see what they can take out or economize.

Skip It?

When my children were younger, one of the things that I skipped often to get in training was sleeping in. I would get up at five in the morning, when my kids were still asleep, and exercise for two hours. I know not everyone is a morning person like I am. If you can't wake up early in the morning, maybe you can give up sleep in the evening either to exercise or to do something else that you are now doing during a time you could exercise.

What can you give up? Television is one of the easiest answers. I like my television, but I have a DVR to record it, so I can watch it on my schedule (usually while training). I don't watch the news. I don't spend time reading the newspaper. I don't often go out for a matinee. I also don't answer the phone during the day unless I have to. I screen my calls. I feel that during the day I need to focus on my work. I don't often go out to lunch with friends. I have rules about how much time I am allowed to spend on the computer using Facebook or other social network- ing sites. I use them as a reward after I finish a task. I keep it down to five minutes at a time.

Another thing that would be on my list of suggested things to skip is the makeup and hair routine. I remember when I was a teenager, an older woman took me aside and explained to me that she knew how to do her hair and makeup in twenty minutes flat. She seemed to think this was such a tiny amount of time to spend on looking beautiful. I'm not saying that people who spend time on beauty are wrong, but that's not my choice. I keep a hairstyle that can be taken care of in less than a minute. I wash and condition it in the shower, then comb it and put it back in a ponytail. I have to be comfortable with people seeing me without makeup on anyway since I do not train or race with makeup on.

My sense of priorities about beauty has trickled down to my kids. When they were younger, my kids had messier hair than their friends, and they didn't get a bath every night, just once a week (before church on Sunday) like my mom did with me when I was a kid. Their clothes weren't as shiny bright as other kids, either, because I didn't clean clothes individually or look for spots to treat. I threw them all in the washing machine and then in the dryer and we have been just fine. Not doing those things gave me time for other things I enjoy, like reading books.

I have always wished that I had a cleaner house, as if wishing for it would make it so, when, in truth, I know that it is really a time commitment I am unwilling to make. So I have skipped the perfectly clean house. I feel guilty sometimes when I see other houses or when guests come to mine. My in-laws are so clean that I am convinced they don't come to visit us often because they cannot stand our house's constant state of disarray. I cannot clean constantly if I want to have time to train, and race, and write, and be a mom. That is one of the trade-offs which I have to remind myself I have decided to make.

Sometimes I go around in the morning and close all the doors to my children's rooms so that I do not have to look at their messes and feel obligated to do something about it. Give yourself permission to do this. You do not have to clean. Your house will not collapse if you give yourself some time to do other things, things that last, unlike cleaning. The dirt will wait for you, I promise.

Another fantastic thing to give up is shopping. I give my kids a yearly clothing budget and we go out at the beginning of the school year. But after that, they can buy clothing online if they have a sudden growth spurt. I don't enjoy shopping, so I don't feel bad giving it up. Still, grocery shopping is a must. If my children need something from the store, it is their job to write it on the list on the refrigerator. I do a big grocery shopping day at the beginning of every month and smaller shopping days each week. Planning a month's worth of meals at the beginning of the month, and making sure that I have on hand at least three meals that I can just throw together at the last minute like frozen ravioli is a huge time saver. I also make double meals. When I make a casserole or lasagna, it's hardly any extra trouble to make a second one. It saves a lot of time on days when the world has gone crazy and I have to be in two places at once and no one has time to go over to McDonalds. It's much healthier too.

As with my house cleaning, this means that I have to be willing to accept a slightly lower level of cuisine. If I have to substitute for something in a recipe my son, Sam, who is an aspiring gourmet, complains. He doesn't cook that way. When he's in charge, he goes to three different stores to get all the proper ingredients. That's his priority, but it's not mine. I want the food to taste decent, be healthy, and keep us going. I admit, if I didn't have to eat three times a day, I wouldn't. I don't love food for its own sake. I hate feeling hungry, but I would be fine with eating one regular meal and lots of healthy snacks each day. If you're not like that and you need to spend hours a day on gourmet meals, this isn't where you're going to find the time, but you can find time somewhere else.

Another thing Americans spend a lot of time on is home repair and decoration. We just don't do that much at our house. We bought a house this time around that we knew we weren't going to have to change. The time before, we bought it for its potential rather than for what it was. I enjoyed redoing the kitchen completely, but after a while it got to be too much and I found that the cost of what we were doing compared to how much we would get out of it when we sold it wasn't much. These days, we pretty much wait for needed repairs and keep the decorating simple. I don't put up new curtains. I don't paint my walls colors other than white. I don't put up wallpaper. I've done it in other houses. I know how to do it, but I don't choose to. I know those things would be nice, but they would make it impossible for me to do other things that matter more to me.

Call in the Reinforcements.

I have a friend who sometimes can't make it to a get together because she has to get her house ready for the cleaners. They come once a month for two hours and she leaves the house and depends on them to do the deep cleaning everywhere she doesn't have time to get to. She also has one of those robot vacuum cleaners that she sets up every morning after the kids go off to school. She swears by these things and says her life is a lot easier because of them. She thinks the cost (two hundred dollars a month) is well worth it. I don't go that far, but whenever I talk to her, I have to admit, I am definitely tempted. She does have to spend time when the cleaners are coming to pick up the normal clutter so that the deeper cleaning can be done, but it forces her to keep clutter in check. More and more women are hiring help to do jobs that they don't prioritize. If you don't have the money for that, may I suggest some other ways to avoid cleaning?

If you have kids, they are a great resource. They help make the mess. It's good for them to do some of the work to help unmake the mess. When kids are small, you can have them do things like put toys into the proper container or pull the quilt up on their beds. They can also be in charge of unloading the silverware from the dishwasher every day or putting glasses on the table for dinner. When my kids were little, I would tell them to go quick and pick up ten things from the living room if we had company coming. Things didn't always get put away in the right place, but it was still helpful. I expected my little kids to help me fold laundry, and by "fold," I mean that they picked up underwear and socks and put them in the right basket. They could also help put away their own clothing.

As they get older, kids can have a lot more responsibility. I used to have a wheel of chores and each kid would have a turn at different jobs like cleaning the sink or vacuuming the front room. Now they have settled on certain jobs that they seem to like more than others. Sage always does the kitchen floor, but she can't stand to do the bathroom. Sam does all the toilets in the house, as long as I remember to get him the cleaner that he thinks is the best for it. I used to also ask each child to help with dinner one night a week, but this has changed over the years. Now I tend to ask kids to help more on an ad-hoc basis. If I am struggling with time, I'll ask for a helper and give suggestions as to what ingredients we have on hand. Sometimes a child will want to do a whole month of dinners if I'm willing to pay them on a per hour basis. I'd rather pay a child to do housework than pay a professional, not because it's more cost effective, but because it teaches responsibility and gives them some good life skills.

I always try to thank my kids for their help and reward them, and I try to be understanding if they have their own crises.

Make a Schedule, but Be Flexible.

I am not one of those people who schedules every minute in an elaborate planner, but believe me, I could be. I'm a little OCD and I like the sense of control that planning a day down to the minute pretends to give to me.

In some ways, I am very strict about my scheduling. I do laundry on Mondays and Thursdays. This actually makes my life a lot easier because I don't have to think every day about whether or not I need to do laundry. I know when I need to do it, and it gets done then. I don't put it off, and therefore I never have children wandering around in a panicked emergency, asking where clean clothes are.

I am strict about bedtime with my kids, because that helps make sure that the whole house shuts down by ten and I can go to sleep at a decent hour. Everyone's lives go better when bedtime is managed strictly. Even on summer break or during the holidays, I don't let them stay up until all hours. And when my kids were younger, I would wake them up early in the morning so that I could make sure they were on the schedule I wanted. Also, if naptimes were synchronized I could get some things done just for me. This may not work for everyone, but it was one of my goals.

I schedule exercise every day, and, depending on what races I'm training for, I carve out an hour to two for it. If there is a reason I can't get in a full workout, I always try to get in a smaller workout. Not just because I'm worried about my training level, but because it makes me feel better. I am a creature of routine, and even if I have to cut my routine short, it still makes me feel that my day is going the right way if it has all the right parts in it. For me, that includes exercise.

Once a week, on Mondays, we have a family tradition of "Family Home Evening." This includes a scriptural lesson, a song, and a prayer. We also hold the all important family scheduling discussion. This is a time for the kids to tell us what commitments they have for the week and what help they will need from us to make those commitments. Matt and I both have an iPhone and we electronically calendar everything. I resisted for years giving my kids cell phones but the oldest four all have them now, and we can text each other freely to make any adjustments to the schedule. I will admit that I sometimes still end up double scheduled for things, or miss an appointment. Scheduling is difficult to do perfectly when you have children involved. I do my best, but like many I am occasionally late picking up my children. My kids have a rule about me buying them ice cream if I'm more than forty minutes late picking them up from school activities.

Sage and Hope, my two oldest girls, have had problems since they've started high school with over scheduling themselves. When I watch them have weeping breakdowns because they haven't had enough sleep and they have homework due the next day, I remind them that when you are working in the real world, you should only schedule yourself up to about eighty percent of what you know you can do each day. The other twenty percent you have to leave open to other people or natural disasters that are surely going to impinge on your time without any warning. It's a good rule for grownups, too. Give yourself a buffer in case of unexpected disaster.

Then always plan some time to yourself every day that is just for fun. Schedule, yes, but accept that the schedule is not the reason for your life. It's supposed to help your life, not make it worse. So be flexible when necessary. If you are truly too sick to work out, then that is what it is. I keep a workout journal and have done for years. I can look back through and see there are days, especially during the Winter, when I simply write in "SICK" and there is no workout that day. I just start over fresh the next day.

Choose a Time That Fits Your Personality and Lifestyle.

The more I train, the more I realize that you have to figure out what works for you, and not just assume that what works for someone else will be perfect for you too. If I tried to do Michael Phelps' swim workout, it would kill me in about ten minutes flat, not make me more like Michael Phelps. It's just going to make me less like me. So, when I see someone decide to make the leap and commit to working out every day, watching calories, and trying to eat healthier food, I cringe if it seems they are committing to something that is so obviously contrary to their personality and lifestyle. Of course, we are all trying to change and become better, but this happens in small steps, not in getting a personality transplant. The reality is, you are who you are. You can become a better you. But you are not going to be someone else.

If you can accept that, then it's time for you to look at your personality and lifestyle and choose what kind of a workout routine is going to be doable for you. Remember, this isn't something that you are going to do for the month of January to make yourself feel better about your New Year's resolution. This is something that you want to able to commit to for the rest of your life. I see little sense in going on a diet for your high school reunion when you are going to gain all the weight back ten months later. Make small changes that you can stick to and you will be better off, both physically and emotionally. You won't beat yourself up about not being able to continue with something that was wildly unrealistic to begin with.

So, first, think about what time of day is the best time for you to exercise. There are different advantages to different times. I've already said that I am a morning person. For years, I could not understand why anyone would exercise at another time than in the morning. Morning exercise makes sense in many ways. If you exercise in the morning, you only take one shower. That saves time. Also, studies show that morning exercise is best because you are at your peak of energy when you have just finished your sleep. Appetite suppression can last for several hours, even until lunch, if you exercise in the morning. And I just think it makes people perkier and happier for the rest of the day. Sometimes it can be easier to have the decision to exercise already made when the alarm clock goes off. You don't try to talk yourself out of it. You just get dressed, go outside or get on the treadmill.

Mornings outside can be a fun time for runners because a lot of other runners are out and runners are often a friendly group. I live in Utah, and the runners who run year round outdoors are hardy. If you like that, get yourself some warm running pants, gloves, hat, and long-sleeved shirts as well as a breathable jacket. You may find a group of runners to go out with or simply enjoy waving to the same group of people as you pass them going in opposite directions. If you like biking, you can get out before traffic on the roads gets too bad or head to a trail before it gets busy. If you don't want to bike outdoors in the winter, even with winter gear to keep you warm, you can buy a trainer and bike indoors all year round. More on that in the tip section later.

If you are a swimmer or want to start swimming, there will be the same group of morning people at the swimming pool you go to. You will get to know them by name or by their stroke pattern. When you are stopped at the side to rest or to change gear, you will likely find yourself chatting with other swimmers. They may give you some helpful tips about swimming, or just encourage you to come back again by their friendly attitude. There are also lots of master swim teams at local pools that you can join. They would be happy to help you learn to swim or to bone up on your skills if you haven't been in the water for a long time.

Morning is a great time, but I am not just an early morning exerciser anymore. I have learned that there are other times of day that can work with my schedule. I now work out midmorning. About three years ago, I invited a friend of mine who wanted to get more fit to meet me at my gym twice a week. She wanted to start at 9:00 a.m. For her, a mother of seven kids between the ages of seven and twenty, right after she dropped the youngest off at elementary school worked best. It turned out to be a wonderful change for me. I find myself still exercising every day at about that same time. Now I wake up between 6:00 and 7:00 in the morning and spend the first couple hours of the day working on my laptop computer upstairs as the kids all get ready for school. I get to participate in the morning banter, make sure that they tell me about anything they need me to do that day, and give them the warm feeling that Mom is there with them.

Some people who work full-time jobs away from home find that lunchtime can be the best time. If you have a gym close to your work, you can bring a bag with shower items and fit in a quick workout and then eat when you get back to work while you're at your desk. A short workout is better than nothing, and there are plenty of lunchtime people at the gym, pool, or outside. I see runners and even more bikers outside during lunch. Sometimes my husband, Matt, will take an extra hour or two for lunch when the weather is cooler in the morning. He goes to work early and then can justify the time off when the sun is up and he will enjoy his workout more. One of the advantages to lunchtime exercise is that it can suppress your appetite. If you have trouble eating too much at lunch or in the early afternoon, this can be one way to deal with it. Even a short burst of exercise in the afternoon while you are struggling with the munchies can stave them off until dinner.

There are days when I fit in exercise at night, though I am not sure whether I should recommend this. If you truly are a night person and you feel renewed energy at night when your kids are in bed, you can try this regularly. I will warn you that studies seem to indicate that, for most people, if you don't get the exercise in first thing, you either won't get it in at all or you won't be able to exercise with the same freshness that you would have in the morning, when you are physically at your best. Still, a lot of triathletes end up having to fit in two workouts a day, and they do one in the morning or at lunch and then another at night. This can be a way to fit in some more exercise time when you have other commitments during the day. If you do want to watch television at night, you can set yourself a rule that you are not allowed to watch unless you are working out while watching. Or you can pay yourself hours of TV for hours of time spent exercising.

The important thing is that you think about what things you will miss the most in your life and you make sure that you try to give up as little of those things as you can while adding your exercise routine in. Do you really need to do the couch potato routine at night as a reward for a hard day? Then a night routine isn't going to work for you. Do you need your coffee before you workout? Maybe you want to do a little later morning workout. Do you need friends to help you get motivated? Then find a friend who is at your level and choose a time that works for both of you.

Multitask and Use 5 Minutes Wisely

Another way to get a little more time into your busy life is to do two things at once. Many women are already doing multitasking like watching TV and folding laundry or helping one child with homework while doing the dishes. I watch plenty of television, but I rarely watch when I am not doing something else. I often watch television while exercising. When I am doing a short workout, I will time the workout to the length of a TV program. If I am watching live television at the gym, I will sometimes watch the TV program while I am going easy, then go hard during the commercials when I don't want to pay as much attention.

You can also multitask in more creative ways. Instead of driving to the grocery store and then heading to the gym, walk or ride a bike to the grocery store. You can jog to the gym and then jog back home to add a few extra miles and this can have the bonus of helping the environment. Hope, my oldest daughter, is convinced that the environment would be completely saved if all Americans just had a bike and we closed all roads to car traffic. People would feel safer biking without cars to contend with, they would save money on gas, and they would get healthier. It would help all around.

If that doesn't work for you, find out what does. It may change from day to day. For years, I could not afford much of anything and I exercised by taking my children out in the stroller for a brisk walk, or by jumping rope while they played, or climbing the stairs in our house that were already there and thus free. I bought old, used Jane Fonda exercise tapes and learned the moves so well I could do them even if I didn't have the tape on. One year I woke up with my early riser, put her in the baby seat on my bike and rode around the neighborhood until my husband and the other kids woke up. In the winter I put my kids on a sled and dragged them around the neighborhood. If we went to a park I did the monkey bars with them to get in a workout for my arms. Sometimes I let babies climb on me while I tried to do sit ups or I would do yoga with my kids climbing on my legs to make it a little harder to hold my balance. You do what you can do. Be creative about it, but make it a priority to be active.

If you only have five minutes, do something with that five minutes. At my house, we keep a set of small weights up by the big television. That way, anytime you want, you can go over and do a few bicep curls or lunges. We have a big poster up, as well, that shows various moves that you can do with an exercise ball. You just have to look up and you can see twenty different ways to get in better shape. Pushups are great exercise. Sometimes with our focus in America on gyms and equipment we forget that some of the best exercises are done with your own body weight, doing real life movements. After all, the point of exercise is, at some level, to make it so that you can continue to live your normal life for as long as possible. You want to be able to carry your own groceries into the house as long as you can, go up and down stairs without assistance, and get in and out of a chair. If all you have is a chair and some cans of food, you can get some good exercise lifting the cans of food in a bag and getting in and out of the chair multiple times.

If you are in bed, you can even do some stretching. I sometimes lie in bed and let my knees bow out to stretch out my inner thigh muscles. Or I lean to the side to stretch out my hips. I will bend over and let my body hang so that I can touch my toes before I go to bed. My mother used to "hang" on her door to stretch out her back. It only takes a few minutes a day and it can make a real difference. The five minutes that you spend playing Angry Birds on your phone or looking on Youtube because you're bored in line at the grocery store can be used for increasing your knowledge of yoga and then practicing it.

Tips on Buying Your Own Exercise Equipment

A great way to save time is to have your own indoor equipment. Then, if you are up in the middle of the night and unable to sleep, you can workout without disturbing anyone and without worrying if the gym is open. You can also much more easily workout with kids, even if they are older. I don't like to leave my kids alone for too long, but if I am downstairs and they know they can come down and ask me a question while I workout, I feel like they are safer.

Exercise Ball

An inexpensive way to get started on toning your body is an exercise ball. A fifteen-dollar investment at your local Wal-Mart or Target, and you will get a ball and a poster with exercises you can do with it to put up on your wall. Warning: Kids love to play on exercise balls. I have to keep mine hidden in my office and remind my kids constantly that they are not allowed to play on it. They can do exercises on it if they get permission, but if the kids use it too much, it tends to get holes in it and deflate. An exercise ball with a hole in it is useless. If you want to use your exercise ball in your family television room, just take it downstairs afterward. Exercise balls are great for core exercises, like crunches and airplane. They are also great for just sitting on. You can kneel or try to stand on them (with support). You can also do lots of other exercises with weights: bicep curls, tricep presses, chest presses, and so on. Then you're activating your core and focusing on a specific group at the same time.

Yoga Mat

A yoga mat is a useful way of carving out a specific space for you to work out on, even if you're not doing yoga. You can tell your kids they have to keep off your mat and show them the line. Also, the grip on the yoga mat is great for doing pushups, which are a staple of my routines because they work on shoulders, arms, and core (abs and back) at the same time. If you have been to a few yoga classes, you can probably make up your own yoga routine. Look up online to find specific moves or get a book for reference. You can also buy DVD's on yoga workouts. I don't like to follow along anyone else's routines, so I tend to make up my own routine, adding in ideas from sports magazines like *Runner's World* or *Cycling* that appear periodically. Some of my basics include planks, downward facing dog, tree pose, advanced tree pose, and cow pose.

Jump Rope

A good jump rope can be a great way to get in some intense aerobic exercise indoors. You need to make sure your ceiling is high enough and your rope is the right length. Also, keep children away while you are doing this. It's a good thing to do during nap time. A mat on the floor will keep your carpet from being damaged, and if you get bored jumping rope, you can skip and do figure eights or learn tricks online. I used to mix jumping rope with stair climbing. One hundred jumps, then up and down the stairs ten times. It was a great way to do interval training without having to go outside or to the gym. It gets your heart rate up fast and keeps it there. You could also mix it up with some weight training.

Weight Bench and Weights

I have a small weight bench in my exercise room that folds up for storage in a corner. I also have a rack and a series of weights.

You can use lots of things for weight lifting, from a gallon of milk to cans of vegetables if you don't have money to buy weights. If you do have money to buy weights, I recommend starting with five and eight pound weights. Workout with those for a couple months and then you'll be ready to move up to a set of ten and twelve pound weights, and your budget won't be so stretched on any given month. With these weights, you can do shoulder shrugs, calf raises, lunges, squats, chest presses, bicep curls and tricep presses. If you have access to an outdoor playground, you can get in some chin-ups, as well, or simply do the monkey bars like your kids do and it will be a great workout for your upper body.

Treadmill

If you are going to buy a treadmill, be aware that you will spend at least one thousand dollars on one you can really run on. If you are OK with a treadmill that is only for walking, you can get away with only three hundred to four hundred dollars. I recommend that you try one out first at a place like Costco or a sports store where they have them set up. You need to find out what size of deck works for your stride. Matt is much taller than I am, so I made sure that he tried out different deck sizes and we got a long one for him to run comfortably. I'm shorter and probably could have gotten away with a smaller deck.

You will also want to make sure that you have the features you care about in terms of speed and incline. Ten miles per hour is probably fast enough for most triathletes who are casual, but there may be some who need a treadmill that will go up to twelve miles per hour. Incline is also great so that you can mimic the terrain of your course. I've never used more than an eight percent incline, but, if you do more walking, you may want to make it more difficult with incline. I never use programs, so those don't matter to me. A treadmill with a built in heart rate monitor is probably more expensive than it is worth. If you want a heart rate monitor, you can buy an inexpensive one for about forty dollars.

Indoor Bike or Trainer

If you are looking for an indoor bike, I recommend spin bikes. They cost more than the magnetic resistance bikes that you see at a lot of cheaper sports stores, up to six hundred dollars versus two hundred fifty dollars, but they are worth it in my opinion. They last a long time, are upright and can be set up to mimic your own road bike or tri bike. But if you are going to spend the money to get indoor equipment, you might as well put as much as you can to getting the best bike you can.

I recommend spending one hundred dollars on a trainer to put your outdoor bike on. You put your back wheel into the trainer and clamp it on. The trainer mainly provides resistance to your wheel while spinning, and you don't really need anything else. Your bike will stand upright on its own while clamped in. After spending money on numerous indoor bike setups, I've concluded the trainer is the best deal for your money. It's also great because it mimics the motion of a race most closely, as you are on your own bike.

Fan and Exercise Mat

You will need a fan in your workout room. I often need two fans in my workout room, one facing me and one behind me. I sweat a lot. I also have an exercise mat (thicker and more in-dustrial than a yoga mat, but about the same size—you can buy them online or at a local store when you purchase any exercise equipment) underneath my bike to catch the sweat so it doesn't get on the floor. It also protects the carpet from spills from my Gatorade bottles. Even in the middle of winter, I will sometimes open the window in our exercise room to add to the air flow. We also keep the vents in our workout room turned off in the winter, so that the room is cooler than the rest of the house. There's no point in paying electricity to heat a room when you're going to open a window or turn on fans to keep it cooler.

Television and Media

I would also recommend strongly that you have a television or computer set up in your exercise room. Matt almost never watches TV. He will turn on a music video station or use his iPod, but I watch a lot of TV. And when I say watch, I mean that I actually listen to it and glance up occasionally. Yes, I miss some things. This means I want a certain kind of TV show to watch, one that doesn't require intense attention or much thought. I once tried to watch David Tennant's *Hamlet* and found that I hated it. Then I watched it again while not exercising and loved it. It was just too cerebral, and that doesn't work when you're biking or running hard. I don't have that much brain power. I just want distraction.

Long series shows with heavy dialog that you can get in bulk are often the best, or miniseries that have multiple episodes so that wanting to find out what happens next makes you wake up in the morning and go workout happily, as a treat for you.

Some shows I have enjoyed watching from beginning to end:

Flash Forward
Star Trek: Enterprise
The Guardian
North and South
Dr. Who
Avatar: The Last Airbender
Leverage
Burn Notice
The Closer
Robin Hood
MI-5
Merlin
Inspector Lynley

CHAPTER 3

STARTING OUT

Some People Are Born Athletes, Then There Are the Rest of Us

I grew up in a very academic family. My parents cared about our grades, not our sports prowess. My dad was a college professor and my mom was a great mom, primarily because she read to us for hours on end. She taught me the value of reading. I made good grades because it was expected of us and because I competed with my siblings on many occasions. I remember that my parents never once came to a swim meet in the three years I was on swim team in high school, but they came to every boring academic assembly I ever got the smallest award in. At a very early age, it was clear to me what mattered to my parents. I got a PhD in German Literature and am now a writer.

Most of my writing friends, when they introduce me to other writers, introduce me primarily as a triathlete who does crazy things like ultra marathons and Ironman competitions. I am able to talk to basically sedentary, intellectual people about things like body motion and sweat in a way that can seem poetic and almost seductive to them. My passion for sports has led many others to train and compete.

I did meet my husband while on the high school swim team. We shared a lane for a year until he graduated. Matt has a lovely, relaxed stroke that comes from years of swimming as a child. I didn't learn to swim until I was a freshman in high school. Though I swam on the high school team for three of my four years, never once did I make state or even win a race. This was devastating for me emotionally since I had spent my last year of high school swimming five hours and ten thousand yards a day (the equivalent of running twenty miles a day in energy burned).

For years after high school swim team I told myself that I just wasn't made to be an athlete. Still, in college, I began a habit of swimming three times a week just to stay in shape. I did a little running in college, as well, but injured myself after a few months and walked with a knee brace under a doctor's orders for several weeks. When I tried running again, I felt pain and worse than that, a clicking sound that reverberated up my spine. I went to another doctor and was told that I would probably never be able to run again, and I gave up. I couldn't even walk much without pain and a clicking sound in my back that Matt could both feel and hear when he walked next to me.

For the next fifteen years, I continued swimming. I got slower year by year as I put on weight and missed workouts with pregnancies. It was when my youngest son, Zach, was about nine months old in 2003 that Matt got a bonus from his work and I decided I would like to use part of it to hire a trainer at our local gym and lose some of the baby fat. I was then about one hundred fifty pounds at 5' 2". Definitely overweight. I spent the next six weeks listing everything I ate in a journal, pumping iron, doing crazy balance stunts on exercise balls, and doing some short running sprints despite my warnings to the trainer that I didn't think running was a good idea. My body composition changed dramatically, though I didn't lose any noticeable weight. More importantly, I felt good. I could move more easily and lift groceries and kids without help.

I had chosen to do indoor cycling classes to avoid knee pain from more high impact sports like running, but instead the knee pain got worse. So, I went to a sports doctor and was ready to be told that I needed surgery on my knees. That is not what he told me. Instead, he said that I needed to do more stretching and that I needed to run. The knee needed more blood flow to it to heal and get stronger and the only way to do that was by running. He recommended that I start very slowly and increase my distance day by day on a treadmill.

I thought this doctor was insane. I remember going home and yelling about him to Matt. My plan after that was to do everything the doctor had outlined and then, when I still had no relief from the pain in my knees, I could go to him and tell him how wrong he had been.

Start as Slowly as Possible

There is no such thing as too slow.

When I was told by the sports doctor to begin running, he said I should start very slowly, and on a treadmill so that it wouldn't hurt my knees. I took his advice quite literally and I ran—.1 miles the first day on the treadmill slowly, and .2 miles the next day. I figured that at this rate, the doctor could not possibly complain that I had tried to go too fast or do too much. I waited for any sign of knee pain, and, to my surprise, did not feel it. I kept working up .1 mile at a time. I did not run every day, but after about three months, I could run six miles at a stretch on a treadmill. Suddenly, I thought the doctor was brilliant. I had thought that I would never run again in my life. I had thought that walking would become gradually more difficult. I expected knee surgery at some point. And I had come to take it as matter-of-fact that I couldn't manage stairs very well. That was eight years ago.

These days, when people tell me that they envy me, that they wish they could be like me, I end up shaking my head, wondering what they are talking about. I am not especially talented. I am not naturally athletic. I don't have a super low heart rate. I don't have an amazing lung capacity. I'm not a Michael Phelps in the water. I don't even have a coach. But I do workout almost every day, and I push myself a little each time. I eat healthy food and not too much of it. I started slow and I've just kept at it. That's the key.

Start Slow and Be Consistent

You can't go out and start training for an Ironman to start with. You can't even go out and run three miles if you haven't been running and not expect to be in enormous pain. When I started, I ran .1 miles, remember? I didn't ramp up fast, either. I went very, very slowly. I had measurable improvements, but they were small improvements.

Start with a goal like exercising ten minutes a day four days a week. This is a goal anyone can do. Even if it's late at night and you've put the kids to bed and are exhausted, you can go out and do ten minutes of walking most days. It will help clear your mind and give you some time to yourself. Once you've been doing that for a month, you can try to increase your goals reasonably. Either choose to do running one day a week or do a minute of running in your ten minute walk. Another reasonable goal is to increase your walk to twelve minutes each day, or do one "long" day each week where you do twenty minutes of walking.

I've never met anyone I thought started with goals that were too small. It's always the reverse. When I'm writing a novel, I have to think about writing one scene at a time. If I think about the whole novel, I am often overwhelmed. But you never sit down and write a whole novel, you actually only write a sentence at a time. And it's far better as a writer to do a page or two a day every day than it is to try to write all day once a month.

The kinds of improvements that you make in athletics are often barely noticeable. If I get one second faster in a three mile workout, I notice that. I write it down in my fitness journal and I consider that something to celebrate. If you are on a machine at the gym, you can pay attention to the number of calories you are burning per hour. Those tell you the effort level you are giving, and you should be trying to improve, one point at a time.

Consistency and very small improvements. That's what makes the difference in improving your physical health. Making big goals and then not achieving them leads to disappointment and frustration, and that leads to giving up. I don't want you to give up or feel bad about yourself. I've had a few friends who set goals to start exercising and then did too much the first day and had to recover for two weeks to be able to do anything again. Then they were afraid to get hurt again. Getting hurt isn't the goal here. Consistency is. You are better off doing a lot less intensity, but doing it every day than going out once a month and killing yourself.

Set Realistic, Healthy Goals

If you want to lose weight, make sure that your goals are realistic and healthy. Look at a standard BMI chart and see what the range for your height is. I don't believe slavishly in BMI charts, but they work as a decent rule of thumb. I tend to weigh a bit on the heavy side of the chart, which I assume is because I have more muscle than other women my size. But I'm in the range. Start there, and don't necessarily think you want to be your high school weight. If you are trying to gain weight but are naturally thin, target the smaller end of the range as a realistic goal for you.

Be aware that those people who lose a quarter pound to a half pound per week are generally the ones who are able to keep it off. This is partly because if you try to lose more weight than that, your body will react as if it is starving and will work against you, lowering your metabolism and trying to conserve energy for a famine. It will send hormones racing to your brain to get you to overeat, and you can only work against those hormones for so long. It is simply more realistic in the long-term for you to change your eating and exercising habits slowly.

If you are trying to gain weight, gain weight by eating healthy food, not by eating junk. Set realistic goals about how many calories extra per day you are going to add to your diet.

Build in the fact that you will sometimes get sick or not feel like working out. That's why you set a goal of four days a week to begin with, not seven. Set goals that you can easily achieve when you are starting out, and you can make the other, more difficult goals later on.

If you have kids, you've probably seen them get discouraged because they think they should be able to do something a grown up can do right away. You've tried to explain to them that it takes years to learn how to cook, or how to draw, or how to make a robot. Give yourself the same advice that you would give to your child.

Accept Your Body Type

You may not be happy if you start working out because you want to look like a model—or like a particular athletic hero/heroine in your life. Everyone has a different body type and while working out and eating healthy will make you look better, it won't essentially change your bone structure.

I'm short and rather sturdy in shape. I'm never going to have long legs. I have had to accept that I don't have much of a waist even when I'm at my best weight. I've been doing this for eight years now and I still don't have washboard abs. I've gone through six pregnancies and the skin is a bit stretched out of shape. My feet and hands are some of my worst features, in my opinion. I don't have slender ankles. I'm not trying to be self-deprecating here. I'm just trying to point out that no one has the perfect body.

You may have a list of things you wish you could change about yourself. That's OK. Some of the things will change, but not all of them will. You are going to have to accept your shape and then make it the best you can. I personally think that a woman with muscles looks great no matter what her shape!

Also, don't be surprised if you don't lose all the weight you think you should after a few months of working out. One of the things that is happening is that you are losing fat and putting on muscle. You won't necessarily see this on a scale, unless you buy a scale that tells you your body fat percentage and even those are based on estimates and assumptions about your gender and your athletic ability. I'm sure my scale never thinks that I have as much upper body muscles as I do and is therefore a bit off. But the trend is the right one.

You don't want to have someone else's body in the end. You want to have your body and make it the best it can be.

Don't Give Up

Please don't give up if you don't see the results you want immediately. This is the thing I see most frequently when I try to help people with their goals. They are excited to work out for about two weeks, and then they lose interest. This is partly because they don't set realistic goals, and therefore get discouraged easily. If your goal is to lose a quarter pound a week and you achieve that goal, you can celebrate and keep going. But if your goal is to lose five pounds the first week and you only lose two, or only a quarter pound, you may give up quickly.

If, in terms of exercise, you have a goal to run a marathon, be aware that this is a long term goal, possibly one or two years in the distance. Keep in mind that your short term goals are the ones you need to celebrate. Say your goal is to walk/run two miles the first week. If you achieve this small goal, give yourself a pat on the back. You've improved a little, and that's all you can expect. If you are able to lift more weight on one machine this week than last week, that's great. If you can do one more lunge, you're doing awesome. If you can bike a half mile more, you are improving.

Also, be aware that you are dealing with a lot more fatigue as you exercise regularly than you were before. You may experience some days when you can't go any farther than you did the day before, or where you feel like you are actually moving backwards. This happens with eating healthy too; you may actually gain weight rather than lose it on occasion. This doesn't mean that you're doing anything wrong. Don't give up or think that exercise or eating healthy just don't work for you. They work for everyone in the long run, I promise!

So if you end up unable to improve on one day, that's OK. Just do your best. Try to finish the distance you wanted to do, but at an easier pace. This happens to me all the time. I get tired for reasons I don't always understand. It could be due to stress about things unrelated to my exercise, hormones, or perhaps I'm coming down with something. Slow down, and keep going.

The first two weeks, most people don't experience too much fatigue, but after that, it can really start to tear at you. Expect that there will be hard days, or even weeks. You are doing something new that you haven't done before and your body takes time to get used to that. Give yourself a real chance to make this work. And remember—it's hard. You shouldn't feel agonizing pain, but fatigue is normal.

The point of exercise is that you are tearing down your muscles. Then your body will build them back up again and you will be stronger. But that process can be exhausting, especially if you aren't used to it. You may feel frustrated hearing runners talking about a runner's high, and imagining that you will never feel a high when you are running because you hate it so much.

Trust that it will happen for you, eventually. When you get used to it and your body is in better shape, you will have days when running or swimming or biking or weight lifting is easy. More than easy even, wonderful—but not if you give up!

Running Tips

How to Enter a Specialty Running Store

The first time I walked into a running store, I was a little nervous. I've seen people walking into a running store for the first time on numerous occasions since then and I see the same nervousness in their eyes. So, let me help you.

When you enter a running store, you will see racks of sporty clothes, running shorts, bras, and shirts. You may have to walk through these in order to get to the back of the store where the actual running shoes are usually located. You may also see other running paraphernalia such as water bottles, water bottle holders, sports gels and other foods, watches and GPS, heart rate monitors, sunglasses, nipple guards, and sunscreen. **Do Not Get Distracted**. Walk toward the running shoes. These are the foundation of your running experience. Everything else is extra.

As you enter a good running store, you may also wait at the door for a few moments, as if in confusion. If the store is especially busy, you may have to walk yourself over to the shoes. I find that if I go during the day, I will usually be greeted by a salesperson. Do not be discouraged by this. I hate salespeople in many situations. When you go car shopping, you cannot avoid a salesperson if you want to drive a car. In a shoe store, I suppose it might feel the same way. You might worry that a salesperson will pressure you and you think you are perfectly capable of looking through the shoes yourself and finding the pair you want and asking for your size. Please do not do this. You don't know what shoes you want. You don't know what size you need. You know nothing. You must allow yourself to be handled by the experts.

A good running store will likely have someone who can put you on a computerized analysis of both your stride and your arch. I have a high arch and so does my husband. We both wear neutral shoes. But the perfect shoes for me are not going to be the perfect shoes for you. A good running store will also explain to you how many sizes up from your regular shoe size you should buy, based on what you are planning to do, how many miles per day or week you will train, and what race you are training for. The longer your race, the larger the shoe you should buy to compensate for the swelling in your feet.

Don't buy online. Even if you know what you think you want to get, don't do it. Support your local running store, who is a leader behind most local races. And you never know when they will surprise you. After having bought the same shoe for about four years, a running store expert recommended a new shoe for me and I have absolutely loved it for the last several months. There is new stuff coming out all the time. So go let yourself be pampered.

The next thing you should know is that a good pair of running shoes will cost you at least one hundred dollars. Don't go to a running store unless you are prepared to spend that much. Don't start running unless you can invest in shoes. If you can't afford that (and believe me, I have been there) you are better off walking. Do not run without the proper shoes. You will injure yourself and hate running, and then you will blame me and tell everyone you know how running is terrible and convince them not to try it.

So, when you are looking for the perfect shoes, it's pretty simple. They are the shoes that feel the best. Good running shoes don't need to be broken in. They are ready to run in the first day. If they don't feel right, take them back. Note: a good running store will let you exchange them. They probably can't sell them again, except as clearance, but they want your business and they will make you happy. If they don't, they're not a good running store.

Now, you need to get proper running socks. You will pay about five dollars a pair for good running socks. They will have NO cotton in them. Cotton socks tend to cause blisters when wet.

With running shoes, and socks, you are ready to begin. You can wear any old sweat pants and T-shirt you want. As you get faster, you will sweat more. Yes, that is a funny reality. The best runners sweat more than the worse runners because they need to in order to get rid of the body heat they create while running. Cotton T-shirts are lousy when wet, but until you are running at full speed for more than forty minutes, a cotton T-shirt is probably fine. All the other stuff is for when you have been at it for more than a year or so. You'll get to know the store employees by name and they'll start giving you information as you need it. Or ask, if you're curious.

A good pair of running shoes lasts for four hundred to five hundred miles. I use two pair of shoes, one slightly older for shorter runs, and one new pairs for runs longer than twenty miles when I'm going to need a lot of support. I also have a pair that I've retired from running that I use to walk around and run errands. Do not use your good running shoes except for running. It will save your legs and your feet. If you end up with a lot of running shoes you can't use, donate them.

Running Technique

Lots of people obsess about running mechanics. I just want to make sure that I'm not doing anything terribly wrong. I'm not planning to go to the Olympics as a runner. I just want to get through the run.

1. Keep your arms at a ninety degree angle. Too acute and you risk shoulder pain. To obtuse and you may not be running as efficiently as you could be.

2. Don't let your arms over swing in front. They should swing back and forth, but not side to side.

3. Keep your stride rate between ninety and one hundred strides per minute at all times, even when running easily. Try to shorten your stride and see how much easier it feels. If you want to figure out what your stride rate is, count each time your right foot lands during one minute. That is your stride rate. For most people, it is seventy to eighty, because most people think that to go faster, they need to take longer strides. The exact opposite is true. If you take longer strides, you actually tend to imbalance your body centering and you will be more likely to have injuries.

4. Your feet should land fairly flatly in the center, but if you land on your heels or toes, make gradual changes, not sudden ones. A good pair of shoes may help with this, or focus a few minutes of each running workout to improving your stride.

5. At a running store, you should be able to find out if you pronate in or out. If you do, get some shoes to help with that problem.

6. Keep your head, neck, and shoulders loose. You don't want to cramp up other parts of your body before you have a chance to work out your legs. Keep your hands loose, not in fists, as you run.

7. When you go up hills, increase your stride rate. Also keep your head steady and imagine yourself being a puppet on a string. Don't lean forward. Don't try to go up a hill at the same pace as you would go on a flat surface. You will go slower, and then you will have the energy to go fast down the hill on the other side.

8. When going downhill, don't take such huge strides that you lose control or that you pound too hard. Let yourself float lightly down the hill.

9. If you are planning on doing a race, try to mimic the course as much as possible in training. Ideally, drive out and actually do the course. If it's too far away, look it up online and see what the incline is like, then set your treadmill to do exactly that. Even though you won't try to go race pace all the time, your brain will feel more used to the terrain if you try to mimic it.

10. Remember that there is a psychological element to training. When I was in high school, the coach would tell us that the person who won the race was the one who "wanted" it the most. I think that's bunk. The person who wins is the person who trains the best. But part of training is the mental aspect, preparing you mind properly. Make up a positive mantra as simple as "You can do it," and repeat it as you run.

CHAPTER 4

FINDING YOUR SUPER POWERS

The Kind of High No Drug Can Give You

Even after I had been running a few months without pain, I still wasn't convinced that this was a lasting improvement in the health of my knees. It might be temporary. I fully expected that the knee and back pain would come back at any moment. So when I saw in a local paper that a marathon was being run the next week, I (foolishly) decided that this might be my only chance to finish a marathon while my knees were still good. Without any training beyond the six miles on the treadmill, I signed up for the Ogden Marathon in May of 2004. A couple of more knowledgeable friends tried to talk me out of it, but I was determined. (Please don't take this as advice. This was a stupid thing to do.)

Eventually, I was convinced to do a walk/run plan where I ran one mile and then walked for one minute throughout the race. I felt great the first ten miles, which were all downhill. Then I started to struggle; it wasn't fun anymore. I tried to keep a person in sight who was going at a reasonable pace and just keep up with that person for one mile. Then I would walk through the aid station and try to get going again with someone else in sight. I remember seeing dozens of people passing me who did not look as though they ought to be able to pass me. One woman had the strangest stride I had ever seen, kind of a hop on one leg and then a twirl with the other. I thought it was weird at the beginning of the race, and then when she passed me at mile eleven, I figured she must be doing something right. Grandparents passed me. People wearing knee braces passed me. Kids who looked like they were maybe eleven or twelve years old passed me. But I kept going. I was determined to finish the race. I had set a goal and I meant to achieve it. After all, I still thought this might be my last chance ever to do a marathon.

At about mile twenty, the race hit Ogden Canyon and was steeply downhill again; this was a lifesaver to me. I looked down at myself while I was running. In addition, the aid stations began to be placed at about the half miles rather than the full miles. I allowed myself to continue to take a one minute walking break at the full mile and then again at the half mile when I hit the aid stations. At about mile twenty four, I felt as if I were in a fog of pain. One of my runner friends had tried to talk to me about signs of injury and how to know if it was time to quit the race. He said that if I started to limp or if my stride changed dramatically, then it was a sign that I had damaged a muscle badly and needed to either walk it or quit. I looked at myself while I was racing and tried to tell if I was lopsided, but even though I was in pain, I seemed to be running OK.

I had told my husband and kids that I thought I would finish in about 4:20. I came to this number based on the assumption that I could continue to run twenty-six miles at about the same easy pace that I often ran my six miles. This was an absolutely ridiculous assumption. I should have added at least two minutes per mile, even if I had trained well. When I hit mile twenty-four, I knew that Matt and the kids would be waiting for me, and that gave me some strength to continue. I honestly did not think about where I was going. I just tried to keep focused on each step. At the time, I had five small children, ages two to ten, and I knew that Matt would be struggling to keep them at the finish line. So I tried to hurry as well as I could.

It also helped enormously that the streets were now downtown Ogden and there were still a lot of people lining them, cheering for the people who came by even if they were strangers. The thought that I was almost there was another help along the way. Just a little while longer I thought, only fifteen more minutes, only fourteen more minutes. I started the final countdown, and actually counted every step of those last two miles, a habit that I have continued to this day when I am struggling. The simple act of focusing on counting numbers helped distract me from the pain I was feeling. My brain doesn't work very well when I am in pain, but I can count to a hundred over and over again. There is also something soothing, almost melodic about the rhythm of my feet hitting the ground and the voice in my mind. A group of cheerleaders doesn't hurt, either.

Finally, I saw the finish line ahead and crossed it making a time of about 4:40. Luckily, they had some volunteers there because I am pretty sure I would have fallen over immediately. I do not know what it is that makes it so that you can finish a running race at an eight minute per mile pace and then as soon as your brain tells your body the race is over, you can't move one inch more. I hobbled toward the woman who was handing out medals, held that medal in my hands, and thought—this is the only marathon I will ever do in my life, so I'm going to keep this medal in a very safe place. I was in agony. I delivered three of my five children at home, without any pain relief, so I knew about pain. This was real pain. Matt came over and had to help me to the car. I was hobbling along very slowly. The kids were running all over the place and I had thought that I would help deal with them, but instead, Matt had to do everything because I was too beat.

We drove over to McDonald's after that and got the kids some food and let them play in the play land. I picked at some French fries not realizing that I was probably massively dehydrated, not to mention in serious need of calories. I learned a lot of things later about long races, but at the time I was ignorant about a lot of the information in sports and human endurance that has been discovered in the last few years.

Now I know that it doesn't matter anymore how sick I feel when I cross a finish line. I take the food that makes me feel least like throwing up, usually bananas and a plain bagel, and I eat it while sitting down and finishing a twenty-four ounce bottle of water. Then I let myself get up again and try to move toward a car. When I got home from the marathon, Matt and I sat in front of the television and watched about ten episodes of 24. My legs went into spasms occasionally. I know now that you have to get up and stretch them a bit and then the spasms stop. But at the time, I could not imagine voluntarily moving. I had to crawl up the stairs.

The next day, it was even worse. I could walk up the stairs, but going down them was impossible. After all marathons, stairs are hard because your leg muscles are shredded. I honestly do not think there is any race harder than a marathon, and this is from someone who has done four Ironmans and multiple fifty mile running races. You can push yourself just hard enough in a marathon that you can really hurt yourself. This particular marathon is mostly downhill, which hurts your quadricep muscles more than your hamstrings. This means that going down stairs is the worst. I went to church that day and saw the few other runners who had done the race hobbling around like me. We congratulated each other on our crazy accomplishment and I thought—I'm going to find something else to do. I have found that my feelings immediately after a race, even a week after, are a poor indicator of how I actually feel about a race. It's like having a baby. Immediately after I had my first child, I called up my mother and told her I could not understand how anyone could ever have another one. How did the human race live on? And my mother, who had had eleven children naturally, laughed and told me that eventually you forget. She's right. I think the human brain actually finds it impossible to store memories of pain in any way that really matters to us. We have to work hard to remember what it was like when we were in pain, and when it's gone, it's gone.

The feeling of accomplishment I had when I finished that first marathon was something that stays with me, even after I have done all the other races I have done. I had told myself for so many years I was no athlete, and now I had done something that few people ever do. I thought only crazy running fanatics did marathons. I thought that was something other people did, and I would never do. It had never even been on the list of things I someday thought I would do, that's how unlikely I thought it was.

I hung my medal up on the wall in my office, along with my scholarship awards from college and my Princeton diploma (written in Latin). That is how proud I was of it. I bought the photos from the race and printed them out. In the aftermath of the race, I talked to runner friends who were astonished at my time, especially given my lack of training. One friend had a sister who trained for a year for the same race and got the same time as me. I shrugged this off as just meaning that I was unusually stubborn.

The reality of the next few months was that I couldn't run for more than two or three minutes at a time. I could walk fine and bike and swim, but running was painful. I asked for help and soon learned the stretches I needed to do to be able to keep running without pain. I still do them regularly and am a firm believer in stretching as a part of my workout routine and physical health. I was lucky I didn't end up needing to go to a doctor after this. Getting injured while training is something you try to avoid, but can't always. There's nothing wrong with going to a doctor if you have persistent pain while exercising. Don't give up. Go to a sports specialist whose goal is to keep you out there rather than someone who gives the easy answer of not running anymore. Yes, there are other forms of exercise, but don't give up what you love unless you absolutely have to. If you've found something that gives you that high, fight for it.

The World Changes When You Believe You Can Do Anything

After that marathon, I was hooked on racing, though I didn't know how long it would last. I signed up for the TriUtah Jordanelle Triathlon, an Olympic distance triathlon (1 mile swim, 25 mile bike, 6.2 mile run), just four months later in August of 2004. I trained on a knobby-wheeled trail bike that Matt had used years before and ended up renting a better bike for race day. Matt and I went down to the race venue the night before, and I had my first experience of swimming in open water; it went fairly well. I did not own a wetsuit at the time. I simply did not have the money to invest in one when I wasn't sure I was going to keep doing this triathlon thing long term. I also wasn't sure I would like swimming with a wetsuit since I was so used to swimming without one.

I could hardly sleep that night for excitement; still we got up in time to arrive at the race about two hours early. I set up my bike and running shoes in the transition area and then got into the water with the other women who were doing the race. I figured I was a strong swimmer, so I placed myself in front. I struggled with the swim, with the feeling of panic in open water, and so many people around me. But once I was a little farther out, I was fine. When I got out of the water, I nearly fell down I was so dizzy. I forgot to take off my goggles and cap and had to run back to put them down. Then I got on my bike and heard from one of the volunteers that I was the fifth woman in the race. It turns out he was wrong. I was more like the tenth, but it gave me a shot of adrenaline, and I started pedaling for all I was worth passing people right and left as we headed up the long hill. I started the run still feeling good and kept passing people.

I finished my first Olympic triathlon in 2:42. I also took first place in my age group, the first time I had ever taken first place in anything athletic in my life.

After that race, my whole life seemed transformed. Everything I had believed about myself changed. For years, I thought of myself as a writer, a sedentary person, a non-athlete, but I couldn't really say that about myself anymore. I wasn't just a jogger or someone who went to the gym for health reasons. I was a triathlete. I was good at this. I had discovered a fierce competitive spirit inside me that I had never known existed. I loved the feeling of racing.

There is a sense of time that is unlike anything else. It is hard to describe, but it is as if the world stops while I am racing. I focus so hard on the event that all my worries and troubles seem to fall away. I don't worry about my kids. I don't worry about my job or the dishes. There is just me and the distance. I don't race because I want to beat other people. I race because I want to beat myself, my old times. I love the feeling that my body can do something that I didn't know it could do.

A stay-at-home mother raising five children was now an athlete. And it suddenly made me wonder what other things I had thought about myself that weren't really true. In 2005, I started taking piano lessons. I have never been musical, but I was driving my daughter to lessons and it occurred to me that there was no reason I couldn't play piano. I've always wanted to, but I thought that it was too late. Years later, I am not a concert pianist, but I can play hymns in church. I can talk with my musical daughter about some of her favorite composers because I have learned to play their pieces.

We often have this idea that when we are a teenager or in college, we decide what we are going to be. We find out then what we are good at. And after that, we spend the rest of our years getting better at that handful of things we have decided we are good at. But there is no reason that we can't continue to learn new things, to find new talents our entire lives. That's what I believe. And I want my children to believe that as well. I have stopped even talking to them about what they are "talented" at and have started talking to them instead about what they want and how many hours it will take to get it. You just have to teach yourself the skills and put in the time necessary to master them.

I am not saying that I'm going to be going to the Olympics anytime soon. I am most likely not a Dara Torres, who surprised us all by winning even in her forties. But I am still improving my times. Some experts in the running world say that most people get slower after age forty and that there are only about five years of real improvement at any age. I think this is bunk and I intend to get better for a long while yet. Check out my tips for getting faster at any age at the end of this chapter.

Racing Isn't for Everyone, But It Might Just Be for You

You don't have to race to get the benefits of exercise. Races can be expensive and there are probably people who are too stressed by racing to enjoy it. But, before you dismiss it easily, consider how useful it can be to have people cheering for you on the sidelines. Think about how you may be able to push yourself harder if you are competing against friends who have signed up for the race— or even strangers you've never met before. Sometimes you find yourself going faster and it doesn't even feel harder.

Racing is a great way to set a goal and put something on the line to achieve it. Saying you want to run five miles at a stretch is a great goal, but signing up for a race and paying for it in advance is another level of commitment. I find that when I pay for something, I tend not to give up as easily. Paying for music lessons for me was a way of proving to myself that I was committed. It meant I practiced every day because I didn't want to be embarrassed at my lessons, and I didn't want to waste money. Races can serve the same purpose. It can be even more of a commitment if you invite friends or family to join you in the race. Then you can all give each other positive pressure to keep up your workout routines.

(Of course, there are times when you won't be able to compete in a race even if you've paid for it. Please be reasonable about dealing with injuries. If you have a stress fracture or have had surgery or some other problem comes up, don't just keep going with the race as usual. You may be able to walk it, but talk to your doctor. You may have to sign up for next year instead. Your family and friends will understand.)

I think racing is also just plain fun. I like to challenge myself to a new race once a year, and then do a few races that I've done in previous years, so I can measure myself against the exact same course. I do have trouble sleeping the night before, but I figure that's stored energy, ready to be released. It can be a great feeling, standing on the starting line, knowing you have prepared yourself well for this moment.

If you involve your family it can be an opportunity for creating traditions and making memories. We have family routines revolving around racing that we all love. One of our rules is that we always go out to eat the night before a race. This is less about carb loading (which you should probably be doing in the whole week before a race) and more about having fun and bonding together. When my husband does a race with his work buddies, they all go out to dinner the night before and bring their families. It's a great tradition. We also go out to eat after the race, though we wait until we're really starved and can do a meal justice. If you have teenage boys, food is particularly important. My son, Sam, says that he races for the free food. I point out to him that all his food is free, but he insists that race food is better. Maybe it is.

There are other fun routines with racing. Getting up early together can feel like a chore, but it's a great time to talk to people you wouldn't have a chance to talk to otherwise. The routine of setting up your race gear on race morning can be fun. You get to talk to other racers, people who have completely different lives than yours, who you would otherwise never meet. You get to see people who have gone through enormous challenges, like cancer, or losing a spouse, or experiencing a terrible crash, and have come through stronger both in body and mind. It can be so inspiring!

After you've finished your race, you can hang around and watch people come in after you. There is something really incredible about watching the last person come through the finish line. Sometimes it's a kid who is doing her first race. Sometimes it's someone who is overweight and trying to be healthy again. Sometimes it's a man in his eighties who looks amazingly good. You never know what will happen at a race, but I've never regretted doing one.

You learn things about yourself in a race that you don't find out in other ways. Are you the kind of person who keeps going after a crash? Are you the kind of person who can deal with a mechanical problem and not get discouraged? Are you the kind of person who will stop and help another racer who is injured? I love racing in part because it feels to me like a bit of life, made more difficult and compressed into a smaller time frame. I learn life lessons all the time in racing, and I love that.

I would say, try a small race to start with. If you are nervous about not liking it, don't tell anyone you're doing it. See how it goes. If you hate it, don't sign up for another one for a while. But try again when you feel more confident and see if you've changed your mind. Or try finding some friends and see if the experience is different if you know other people there.

Be reasonable in your expectations, but also know that once you have done a race, you may find your whole life has changed, and that you are transformed the way that I was—inside and out.

How to Write Your Own Training Plan

It's not hard to make your own training plan tailored to your specific race and your level of fitness. Make sure you start slowly and that you make a plan that works for your commitment level. I have some sample plans listed below, but you can easily make a custom plan for any race you want to try, though I recommend starting with a short race to begin and moving up in distance from there. Ironman training shouldn't start until you have been exercising regularly for a year. For marathon training you need about six to eight months minimum of running behind you before beginning marathon training.

Choose a Date

To make your own training plan, you need to make up a calendar starting with the day of the race you are targeting.

Make a Long Day

Whatever your race distance is, from 5k to an ultra marathon, find a day you can go long. Saturday is the day that works for me, but whatever day it is, make it a regular date. Long workouts give you enormous benefits in terms of easy aerobic training, and it should feel easy, so go a lot slower. If you have a race 10k or under, you should work up to a longer distance for your Saturday or "long day." Plan on your long day being at a very slow pace, about two minutes slower per mile for running than your actual race.

How Many Days Can You Train?

I have done training plans for races up to Ironman distance or even fifty mile running races with only four days a week training about an hour a day on weekdays: Monday, Wednesday, Friday, and a Saturday long day. Be realistic about what you can do.

My husband can't train five days a week because of his work schedule. When I was doing Ironman training, I didn't train on Sundays. That's my holy day and even though all the training plans I ever saw had a Saturday/Sunday block, I didn't do it that way. If you can only do thirty minutes three days a week, pick a shorter race, make that your commitment, and do it.

Figure Out Your Peak Week

For Ironman training, this is five weeks before the race day. For marathoners, it is four weeks before. For a 10k or 5k, I would say two weeks before. Your peak week distance should be close to your race distance for a marathon or a triathlon (about twenty-two to twenty-three miles). For an Ironman or a half Ironman, you will need to do two long days one after the other. You will do a little more than half race distance on the bike one day, and you will do another half of the race distance the second day, combined with a thirty- to sixty-minute run. As you taper, you will decrease the distance for each day, but you will continue to have two long days blocked together. Look at the training plan and this will make more sense.

Lead Up To Your Peak Week With Slow Increases

Add no more than ten percent per week to your overall distance. That means if you start with one mile, it's going to take a while to move up to twenty miles. If it is more than four months until your peak week, you will need to plan in several down weeks. You build up for four to five weeks, then take it easy for a week, then begin to build again.

Do one Day a Week of Hard Speed Work

Many training plans have two days a week for this, one for shorter intervals, one for a longer tempo workout. I'm getting old, so I can usually only manage one a week. Do a regular warm up and cool down. Intervals are like doing four quarter-mile sprints with a quarter mile to a half mile of walking or easy jogging in between. A long tempo would be two miles warm up, a two- to four-mile run at a hard pace similar to your race pace, and then a two-mile cool down.

Do a Brick Workout Once a Week

A "brick" workout is one in which you move from one discipline to the other seamlessly. You don't need to do a long swim workout in order to get the feeling of what it is like to get on the bike afterward, but you need to get used to doing that to succeed in transition. Do a short warm-up and a short cool down, two to three minutes, if you need to save time. Then do some intense work for thirty minutes to fifty minutes.

Schedule a Taper After Your Peak Week

Continue the same format as your earlier weeks, but cut ten to twenty percent each week. Keep doing some hard workouts, but not for as long. The point here is that you don't want your muscles to forget what race intensity is, but you want them to be rested up.

If you taper too much, you may end up with a slower race pace than you want. Ask my husband. He made this mistake with our fifty-mile run in 2009. He thought if he followed the schedule up to peak week, he didn't have to worry about the rest. This was a big mistake. He stopped working out for almost three full weeks before the run and then ended up having to walk almost the entire race. He is still disappointed in himself for the result.

Plan Some Yoga and Stretching Into Your Schedule

If you can do even ten minutes twice a week, you will be able to count on fewer injuries. If you can't find a class, get a video at home and figure out some of the workouts, then do it in the evening or during a lunch break. This doesn't need to be connected to another workout.

Plan 20 Minutes each Week Weight Lifting/Core Workout

Do three sets of ten reps each, of four or five different kinds of exercises. Three sets of ten push-ups is great, with sit-ups, lunges, and squats, it's a full workout. Or you can do circuit training at the gym and do a set of ten on each machine, moving to the next without a break to maximize your time. I tend to do the minimum weight lifting during racing season in the summer and more in the winter as it becomes less pleasant to be outside. Weight lifting is also a great way to lose weight if you are watching your calories closely. You don't feel as hungry after lifting, and your body can get nicely sculpted. But when you are doing intense weight training, cardio work has a tendency to get left a little on the back burner. That's fine. Doing different cycles of training is a great way to keep things fresh.

Sample Training Plans

Here are some plans you can begin with. If you have extra weeks, I would recommend that you begin slowly and then use the chart, rather than adding more intense workouts in the middle. I don't mean for anyone to follow these plans slavishly. If you need to, switch days around or modify it as you need to. Just as a warning, however, the more you change it, the less useful the plan may end up being.

Key:

- WU = Warm up (for 5 minutes unless otherwise stated)
  When you are warmed up, you should feel your muscles are warm, but you shouldn't be short of breath.
- CD = Cool down (for 5 minutes unless otherwise stated)
  When you cool down, you should slowly decrease your speed after each minute, until the last minute is very easy, walking or similar pace.
- EZ = Easy, so you could easily hold a conversation while exercising.
  For reference as you use the charts, see chapter three for swim drills, chapter seven for tips on bike technique, and chapter three for tips on running technique.

I do not write in WU and CD on every square in the plans. You should always start with a warm up and always end with a cool down.

5K Training Schedule

Week	Monday	Tuesday	Wednesday	Thursday	Friday	Saturday
1	Walk/run 2 miles, 1 minute running every 5 minutes		Walk/run 2 miles, 1 minute running every 5 minutes		Walk/run 2 miles, 1 minute running every 5 minutes	Walk 3 miles total, no running
2	Run ½ mile straight through. Rest 5 minutes. Run ½ mile straight through again		Walk/run 2.5 miles, 2 minutes running every 5 minutes		:30 weight training and/or stretching	Walk 4 miles total, no running
3	Walk/run 2 miles, 3 minutes running every 5 minutes		Run 1 mile straight through. Rest 5 minutes. Then run 1 mile straight through again		Walk/run 2 miles, 3 minutes running every 5	Walk 4.5 miles total, no running
4	:30 weight training and/or stretching		Walk/run 3.5 miles, 3 minutes running every 5 minutes		Walk/run 3.5 miles, 3 minutes running every 5 minutes	Walk 5 miles total, no running
5	:30 weight training and/or stretching		Walk/run 4 miles, 3 minutes running every 5 minutes		Walk/run 4 miles, 3 minutes running every 5 minutes	Walk 5.5 miles total, no running
6	Walk 1 mile. Run 2 miles straight through. Walk 1 mile.		Walk/run 5 miles, 3 minutes running every 5 minutes		:30 weight training and/or stretching	Walk 6 miles total, no running
7	Walk/run 3 miles, 3 minutes running every 5 minutes		Walk/run 3 miles, 4 minutes running every 5 minutes		Walk 1 mile, run 1 mile, walk 1 mile	Walk 4 miles total, no running
8	Walk/run 3 miles, 2 minutes running every 5 minutes		Walk 2.5 miles, no running			Race day

Walking a Half Marathon in
12 Weeks

Week	Monday	Tuesday	Wednesday	Thursday	Friday	Saturday
1	Walk 2 miles		Walk 2 miles		:30 weight lifting and/or stretching	Walk 4 miles
2	Walk 2.5 miles		Walk 2 miles		:30 cross-training on a bike or in pool	Walk 4.5 miles
3	Walk 2.5 miles		Walk 2.5 miles		:30 weight lifting and/or stretching	Walk 5 miles
4	Pick up the pace: Walk 2 miles, but 2 minutes faster than in week 1		Walk 3 miles		Walk 3 miles	Walk 6 miles
5	:30 weight-lifting and/or stretching		Walk 3.5 miles		Walk 3 miles	Walk 7 miles
6	:30 cross-training on a bike or pool		Pick up the pace: Walk 3 miles, but 3 minutes faster than week 5		Walk 4 miles	Walk 8 miles
7	Walk 1 mile easy, then walk 2 miles as fast as you possibly can, walk 1 mile easy again to cool down		Walk 3 miles		:30 weight-lifting and/or stretching	Walk 9 miles
8	Walk 4 miles		Walk 4.5 miles		Walk 4 miles	Walk 10 miles
9	Walk 3 miles		Walk 3 miles		:30 cross-training on a bike or in a pool	Walk 11 miles
10	Walk 3 miles		Walk 2.5 miles			Walk 13 miles
11	Walk 2.5 miles		:30 cross-training on a bike or in a pool		Walk 4 miles	Walk 6 miles
12	Walk 2 miles		Walk 2 miles			Race Day

Run a Half Marathon in 12 Weeks

Week	Monday	Tuesday	Wednesday	Thursday	Friday	Saturday
1	Weights :30	Run 4 x ¼ mile sprints, with ¼ mile walking rests inbetween	Cross-training :30	Run 2 miles	Run 2 miles	Bike :20 Run 3 miles, 1 min walking after every mile
2	Weights :30	Run 3 x 1/2 mile sprints, with 1/2 mile walking rests inbetween	Cross-training :40	Run 2.5 miles	Run 2.5	Bike :30 Run 3.5 miles, 1 min walking after every mile
3	Weights :30	Run 4 x ¼ mile sprints , ¼ mile walking rests inbetween	Cross-training :40	Run 2.5 miles	Run 3 miles	Bike :30 Run 4 miles, 1 min walking after every mile
4	Weights :30	Walk 1:00 (4 miles)	Cross-training :40	Run 3 miles	Run 3 miles ½ mile running ¼ mile walking	Bike :30 Run 5 miles, 1 min walking every ¾ mile
5	Weights :30	Run 3 x3/4 mile sprints with ½ mile walking rests inbetween	Cross-training :40	Walk 1:00 (4 miles)	Run 2.5 miles	Run 6 miles, 1 min walking every mile
6	Weights :30	Run 4 x ½ mile sprints, with ¼ mile walking rests inbetween	Cross-training :40	Run 3.5 miles	Walk 1:00 (4 miles)	Run 7.5 miles, 1 min walk after every mile
7	Weights :30	Walk 1:00 (4 miles)	Cross-training :40	Run 4 miles	Run 4 miles ½ mile running ¼ mile walking	Run 9 miles. 1 min walk after every mile
8	Weights :30	Run 4 x ¼ mile sprints, with ¼ mile walking rests inbetween	Cross-training :40	Run 4.5 miles	Run 4 miles	Run 10 miles, walk :45 sec after every ½ mile
9	Weights :30	Walk 1:00 (4 miles)	Cross-training :40	Run 4 miles	Run 4.5 miles	Run 12 miles, walk 1 min after every mile
10	Elliptical :40 Weights :30	Run 3 x ½ mile sprints with ¼ mile walking rests in-between	Elliptical :40 Weights :30	Run 4 miles	Run 5 miles	Run 8 miles, 45 sec rest every ¾ mile

| 11 | Elliptical :40 Weights :30 | Walk 1:15 (5 miles) | Elliptical :40 Weights :30 | Run 3 miles | Run 5 miles, ½ mile running ¼ mile walking | Run 6 miles, 1 min rest every mile |
| 12 | Elliptical :40 Weights :30 | Run 2 x 1 mile sprints, ½ mile walking inbetween | Run 4 miles | Run 4 miles | Run 4 miles | Race Day |

Sprint Triathlon

Week	Monday	Tuesday	Wednesday	Thursday	Friday	Saturday
1	Swim :20 (10 min drills, then a 500 without stopping)	Bike :30 (WU 5 min, Intervals hard 4 x 3 min with 2 min recovery, CD 5 min)	Swim :20 (10 min drills, 5 x 100 hard)	Run :30 EZ	:30 weight training and/or stretching	Bike :45 EZ
2	Swim :30 (10 min drills, 700 without stopping)	Bike: 40 (WU 5 min, Do 30 min 200s hard with 2 min rests, then CD)	Swim :20 (10 min drills, 500 alternate one 50 hard then one 50 easy) Bike:15	Run :30 (WU 1 mile 2 x ½ mile hard with ½ recovery, CD)	Swim :20 (10 min drills, 5 x 50 hard, with lots of rest between)	Bike :25 Run :15 EZ
3	Swim :20 (1000 without stopping) Bike :40 EZ	Bike :30 EZ Run :20, (First 10 min EZ, next 10 min at race pace)	Swim :20 (find a lake or reservoir to try an open water swim EZ)	Bike :30 EZ	Run: 40 EZ, but finish strong (last 5 minutes at race pace)	Bike 1:00 EZ
4	Swim :20 EZ Run :20 at race pace	Bike :20 EZ	Swim :30 (10 min drills, 2 x 500, second one faster than first)	Run :30 (WU 1 mile, Run 1 mile at race pace, CD 10 min)	Run :40 EZ	Bike :30 Run :20 EZ
5	Swim :20	Bike: 40 (WU :10, 2 x 10 min hard, with 5 recovery in-between, CD)	Swim :30	Run :35 (WU 1 mile, Run 2 miles at race pace, CD 5 min)	Run :40 EZ	Bike 1:10 EZ
6	Swim :30 (WU, 10 min drills, 1500 straight through, CD)	Bike :45 Go at race pace for 1 min. out of every 5 min	Swim :20 EZ (Open water—make sure you can get in and out of your wetsuit—count strokes to get a sense of distance)	Run :30 Keep increasing pace every five minutes until end	Bike :45 WU :10, :30 at race pace, :5 CD	Bike :40 Run :30 EZ

| 7 | Swim :20 At race pace Bike :20 EZ (make sure your transition between the two happens as soon as possible to mimic race conditions) | Bike: 30 EZ | Swim :30 (10 min drills, 1000 without stopping) | Run :30 (WU 10 min, one mile at race pace. CD 10 min) | | Bike :40 EZ |
| 8 | Swim :20 (10 min drills 500 EZ) | Bike :20 EZ | Swim :20 (10 min drills, 5 x 50 hard, with lots of recovery inbetween | | | Race Day |

Blank Plan

Here is a blank plan for you to add your own specifics using the guidelines laid out above.

Week	Monday	Tuesday	Wednesday	Thursday	Friday	Saturday
1						
2						
3						
4						
5						
6						
7						
8						
9						
10						
11						
12						

10 Keys for Getting Faster at 40 or Any Age

1. Deal with your nerves. For me, dealing with nerves has also meant accepting that feeling nervous is part of the process, and that my body is storing up energy to release the moment that the gun goes off. After the race starts for most people, the nervousness is gone.

2. Eat well, before, during, and after working out or racing.

3. Sleep well, as much as you possibly can. I used to think I could get by on five to six hours of sleep a night. I can get by with that, but it is not optimum. Naps count too—take one when you can.

4. Learn to take breaks when necessary. When it isn't racing season, keep exercising, but at a reduced level. Also, take a few days off here and there.

5. Go slow on long workout days—slower than you think you should go, and then even slower than that.

6. Race less, optimally once a month or less. Don't follow the temptation to race just because friends are racing.

7. Do weight-lifting and stretching regularly. This will help prevent injuries.

8. Get some help. If you can afford to hire a coach or a personal trainer, even for a little while, it is worth it. A trainer can help you avoid making mistakes. If you can't afford this, consider joining a triathlon club so that you can get tips from other members.

9. Get the proper equipment for your event. You can get inexpensive equipment if you have to, but don't try to do a race without the proper gear. It will be frustrating and possibly dangerous.

10. Have positive self-talk after a race, even if you did not meet all your goals.

CHAPTER 5

YOUR BODY IS A MACHINE, NOT A MANNEQUIN

t's essential that once you have worked out a plan to follow to achieve your goals, you keep in mind some important principles about how your body works. Although we live in our bodies, we sometimes seem surprised to discover that there are rules to keep a body operating properly, just like there are rules to keep any other machine operating properly. If you have a computer, you expect that the computer needs daily electricity to keep operating. If you have an oven, you know it needs gas or electricity to continue to work. We understand there are lots of unexpected glitches that will require a maintenance check by an expert. The more complicated the machine, the more expensive the expert. And your body is an awfully complicated machine.

The thing is, if you keep running your car on the cheapest gasoline and you never take it in for maintenance, what do you think will happen? It will have problems. The problems may be different for each car. One car may start stalling in the middle of traffic. Another car might make great plumes of smoke as it runs, or simply not start at all. I suppose you might even convince yourself that it's OK, that you can learn to live with these "inconveniences" and you keep living your life the same way.

I see a lot of people give up on running because they get an injury of some kind. Certainly there are injuries after which a doctor will demand that you stop running. I wouldn't tell you to ignore your doctor. But if you feel pain while running, you can most often figure out how to deal with it. You wouldn't accept that a car could only drive you three miles without stopping, so why should you accept that from your body if you don't have to? Your body needs you to pay attention to what it is telling you. A sore muscle is a message to you, and it isn't usually a message to quit. It is a message to do something differently. If you feel winded while you run, that doesn't mean your body can never run. It probably means that you have to build up to it. If you feel like you are drowning in the swimming pool, that doesn't mean you can never be a swimmer. It only means that you need to get the right equipment and some lessons, just as you would make sure your car would have a different oil mix in the winter or in a different climate.

Think about other living creatures and how their bodies work. Their needs are not so different from us humans. Owners of animals as pets take their pets out for regular exercise. They make sure that their pets get healthy food. They try to keep them away from eating things that might be harmful for them, not because they want their pets to look "hot," but because they want them to be happier. But the point is we need to exercise and to eat the right food to be happy just as any pet does. The better your machine runs, the better your mind will work too. You will find that you are happier, deal better with others, and are more efficient at your job. You will probably sleep better too.

Think About What Your Body Can Do, Not What it Looks Like.

This summer Sam started to enjoy slapping me on the thighs and saying, "You have huge thighs, Mom." I could have been offended by this, but instead I decided that I really liked him to think of me, at 5' 2" as big. What is really wrong with being big? Big can be strong for a man or a woman. So I told Sam I knew I had big thighs. One day we even got out a measuring tape and I discovered that my thighs are actually an inch wider around than his are. So that's part of the reason that I do well on a bike. I'm not as good at running, I think because runners tend to have smaller frames and the weight of big thigh muscles slows them down since when you run you have to propel all of your weight. While on a bike, your weight is supported and having big muscles there (to a certain level) is an advantage.

I also have big shoulders and arms for a woman because of my swimming and weight training. When I go to the gym, I see men almost always trying to build their upper body and women almost always trying to build their lower body and abs. Trying to figure out how to make your body into some weird ideal that is both buxom and thin (for women) or sculpted (for guys) is making us all crazy. There is nothing wrong with a woman with a well-defined back and shoulder area. My kids have learned that when they want to make me happy, they should tell me that I'm strong or tough, not that I look pretty.

I have friends who are small and who wish they could gain weight. I have friends who wish they could lose weight. Most Americans do tend to be overweight, but our obsession with being thinner doesn't seem to be helping us. I sometimes think that if we would stop trying to lose weight we would all be better off. If instead we spent our time thinking about what food really made us feel good and made us better able to function, our bodies would naturally be in better shape.

I have recently started going to Cross-Fit, a gym that focuses more on weight-lifting. If you went, you would be astonished to see the variety of shapes. Some of the women are thin, tall types who look like they might be models. Some are average height, but bulging with muscles and can do incredible things. Some look overweight, but are actually carrying enormous muscles under a thin layer of fat and can out bench press me easily.

All of these body types are doing what they are meant to do. They look great because they feel great, and because they are proud of their bodies. It isn't about the number of inches around their waist or what size jeans they can fit into. At Cross-Fit, everyone writes on the white board what weight they lifted or how many repetitions of an exercise they could do. That's the focus—the end result of having a body that is fit—and that is the way it should be. Ultimately, we want to be able to keep living as well as we can for as long as we can, hopefully into our eighties and nineties without assistance if we can manage it.

Get a New Scale

To understand our fitness, we need to do more than just look at numbers on a typical bathroom scale.

I had a neighborhood friend I was talking to about exercise one day. She told me she had tried jogging for some time. Over four months, she had worked up to jogging four miles a day, and then she gave it up. When I asked her why, she said it was because she had lost about three pounds the first month, and then she didn't lose any more weight. I was aghast at this. She didn't lose weight? That's why she stopped exercising? If losing weight is the only reason you exercise, then it is true that you might not get what you want because you may in fact be adding muscle as you lose fat and a simple weight scale will not show that.

If you are someone who is frustrated because you have tried exercising and you haven't seen any weight loss and you feel like it's useless, let me suggest that you should measure your progress in a different way. First of all, you can get a scale that measures not only your weight, but your body fat. These scales are not one hundred percent accurate. They make assumptions about your distribution of fat especially in the upper body, but they will tell you about trends. If you are not losing weight but your body composition is improving, this kind of scale will reflect that.

A lot of people (and their doctors) focus on the government's body mass index (BMI) charts or calculator. These are meant to be a general rule of thumb for describing the average ratio of height to weight and danger zones of being "overweight" or "underweight."

If your doctor has already shown you this chart or calculator and told you that you are overweight or obese, but you didn't understand what that meant, I hope I can help explain it here. BMI is simply a way of describing the ratio between your height and weight. Tall, thin people will have a very low BMI and shorter, heavier people will have a much higher BMI. In this case, a lower score is usually better (though being in the underweight category can have its own risks.)

According to the CDC, having a BMI over twenty-five is generally considered a sign of excess body fat. The CDC does admit that women will have a higher BMI than men at the same weight as well as a higher amount of body fat even at a healthy weight. Also, as people age, they often tend toward higher body fat. In fact, the chart itself has its limitations, including people like body builders who have a higher than average amount of muscle weight, and therefore will not have the dangerous levels of body fat which the BMI charts are meant to warn against.

The CDC says, "It is also important to remember that weight is only one factor related to risk for disease," and that, "the National Heart, Lung, and Blood Institute guidelines recommend looking at other predictors," which they list as waist circumference and other risk factors such as high blood pressure or physical inactivity.[1]

If you can decrease your waist circumference and your blood pressure and increase your daily physical activity, this may actually matter more than your BMI (though for most people doing these three things will naturally make your BMI decrease). If you feel frustrated that you haven't seen weight loss when you've tried to exercise before, reconsider what you are using to measure improvement. Weight may not be the best marker of your health. Try measuring blood pressure at a local pharmacy and measuring your waist.

Another friend of mine worked out with me for several months and was frustrated because she hadn't seen weight loss. But when she went to her doctor and he told her that her cholesterol had dropped thirty points, she learned exercise is not just about losing weight. "Whatever you are doing," he said, "keep doing it."

In accordance with my friend's experience, doctors at the University of Texas Health Science Center studied the effects of exercise on cholesterol levels. Their test used three groups of women: long-distance runners, joggers, and inactive women. They discovered that the long-distance runners had a far lower LDL, what we know as bad cholesterol level, than could be explained by any difference in food intake, and that even accounting for differences in body fat, the most active women had far higher HDL, or good cholesterol levels.[2]

You have to get a blood test at a doctor's office or hospital to find out your cholesterol level, but if you are waiting for your next regular checkup for that, resting heart rate may also be an excellent way of measuring your risk of heart disease. A group of doctors reporting in The Canadian Journal of Cardiology in May 2008, looked at over thirty-eight studies using 180,000 people in many different countries. The studies showed that as you increase your exercise, your resting heart rate will go down. And resting heart rate is an excellent "predictor of clinical events," meaning diseases ranging from cancer to hypertension (high blood pressure), to cardiac arrest, and heart disease. The article itself explains in some detail why a lower resting heart rate has benefits to your heart function including endothelium stress being lowered. But basically, it means that lowering your resting heart rate through exercise is of at least equal benefit to many of the drugs that are given to help patients deal with heart disease and high blood pressure.[3]

You can measure your own resting heart rate easily right at home. The way to do this is to remain lying down for several minutes when you wake up in the morning. Then put a finger to your neck or your wrist and find your pulse (or use a heart rate monitor if you have one). I usually look at my watch for six seconds while counting beats and then multiply the number of heart beats in that time by ten. My resting heart rate is usually somewhere in the forties, which is good, but there are endurance athletes better trained than I am who have a resting heart rate in the thirties. Be aware that as soon as you even sit up and certainly when you stand, your heart rate will increase. And after you have been awake for several hours, the same is true, so don't do this test in the afternoon or late at night and always lie as flat as you possibly can. Resting heart rate is a great, cheap way for you to measure your own fitness level.

If you think that you are getting older and that you just can no longer be fit, you are wrong. Deborah Kotz of the Boston Globe writes about a new ground breaking study performed at Tufts University that shows even elderly people can successfully fight what may seem like a normal loss of muscle mass and capacity simply by doing regular weight-lifting.[4] And lifting weights twice a week is the government's new recommendation for adults over age thirty-five, according to the CDC.[5] If you want to continue to have greater mobility as you age, lifting weights is a great way to do this.

A 2011 study in *The Physician and Sportsmedicine* has shown that male and female triathletes (a particularly good data point because triathlon requires a wide range of muscles rather than a running-only strategy) who were forty and older were able to preserve muscle mass far beyond their counterparts who were less active.[6]

The conclusion here is that many aging adults lose muscle mass because they aren't using it, not because it has to be a natural part of aging.

If you are interested in more information about how to stave off the effects of aging, the book *Younger Next Year* by Chris Crowley and Henry Lodge is a great resource for nutrition and exercise and other lifestyle choices that will help you live longer and feel younger into your eighties. You can also visit their website: http://www.youngernextyear.com/.

Another idea to measure your increased fitness is to measure what you can do, not just what you weigh. If you are weight lifting, you can keep records of how much you can lift and how many reps you can do. If you can do one more rep this week than last week, you are improving. You are getting stronger and that means you are going to live longer and enjoy a better life. You can use a notebook to keep track of your improvement. Look back at your past workouts often, because sometimes early gains come quickly and then you may feel like you are plateauing for months at a time. You are still improving, but just more slowly.

If you are doing mostly cardio work at the gym, try looking at the calories you are burning using an exercise machine that counts them. If you don't have one that measures calories or you exercise outside, you can get a heart rate monitor that will estimate calories burned. This will help you measure how much effort you are putting into a workout, then you can increase your effort day by day. The longer your heart can keep your body moving at an aerobic level, the better your overall health will be and the longer you will be able to continue to remain mobile in your older years.

With a committed exercise routine and healthy eating, you can stay healthy longer and stop many of the effects of aging. Some people tell me that I look young enough to pass for a teenager, especially when I'm with my own teens. I have no desire to go back to my teen years, but I think what they mean is that I still look fit. And I feel great. I am actually faster than I was as a teen, and I think I'm healthier. I can do things now that I could never do then, including pull-ups, handstands, and weight-lifting snatches with a bar. In fact, Sam, my fifteen-year-old sometimes says that he finds it embarrassing that his mom runs faster than he does. Well, I hope this gives him some motivation to work harder, and also a different idea of how aging has to work for him when he's older.

Eat to Fuel a Healthy Lifestyle

For some reason these days, women and men are continually looking to cut calories out of their diet, particularly carbohydrates. But there is nothing wrong with carbs. Eating carbs is good for you. The Paleo Diet, the Zone, and even the Atkins Diets are still popular, and they all emphasize cutting carbs and eating more protein. But the best scientific studies I have seen link high protein consumption—common in a normal American diet—with many health concerns, including cancer, diabetes, osteoporosis, and heart disease. About six years ago I read *The China Study*, a book by father and son team T. Colin Campbell, a Professor of Nutritional Biochemistry at Cornell University, and Thomas M. Campbell II, who is a physician. They looked at mortality rates and diet around the globe. The long list of diseases that are related to a higher animal based diet convinced me to go vegan immediately. I have since slid back a little and have re-introduced milk products and eggs into my diet occasionally. While focusing on getting more protein and less carbs may cause temporary weight loss, this type of diet is proven to increase your risk of cancer, diabetes, Alzheimer's, and MS. On the other hand, a plant-based diet can lower your risk of all these diseases. I'll stick with plants.

Carbohydrates are your main source of energy. As a human machine, you cannot do cardio workouts well without carbs. In *Sport Nutrition, Second Edition*, Asker Jeukendrup, PhD, and Michael Gleeson, PhD, synthesize various studies done in sports to prove that drinking sugar for workouts of longer than forty-five minutes maintains better blood glucose and carbohydrate oxidation. It may also spare glucose in the liver and the muscles. Tennis players who took in sugar while exercising also had improved stroke, so muscle coordination and brain processing may also be improved by sugar ingestion.[7]

In addition, an article in the *Los Angeles Times*, August 31, 2009, summarizes a brain scan study performed in the Netherlands by Paul Smeets, a neuroscientist at University Medical Center Utrecht. Smeets used a technique called functional magnetic resonance imaging (fMRI) to measure how the brain reacts to real sugar verses artificial sweeteners to show that the brain has little response to artificial sugars, even when the test subjects thought they were ingesting real sugar. When the brain sensed real sugar in a drink, even if it wasn't swallowed, it stimulated increased physical activity.[8] So, taking in some real sugar or carbs while exercising hard can actually improve your performance, and ultimately lead you to exercise harder, which will burn more calories.

Yes, processed carbs have been stripped of a lot of nutrients, and you can avoid those. But healthy whole wheat bread and some pasta is not going to hurt you if you eat them in moderate amounts. If you want to know what a moderate amount is, check calories and overall daily carbohydrate intake online at calorieking (http://www.calorieking.com/foods/) or myfitnesspals (http://www.myfitnesspal.com). If you plan to exercise, you are going to need to fuel that exercise before, during, and after. The key is to fuel it the correct way.

You need carbohydrates to restore lost energy supplies, and you need protein to rebuild. Nancy Clark of the American Dietetic

Association and the American College of Sports Medicine recommends a post-workout recovery meal with a ratio of four grams carbohydrates to one gram protein (or possibly as much as two to one) to be consumed within thirty minutes of the workout for maximum efficiency.[9] Chocolate milk happens to be a perfect ratio of four to one carbs to protein, but if you look at the nutrition details, you can manage the same ratio with yogurt and fruit or other snacks. Most people prefer to drink their recovery calories so they can get them down quickly and head for the showers, and this may be one of the few cases where I think consuming a quick recovery shake product may be wise. Remember, you should take in this four to one ratio carbs to protein within thirty minutes of finishing your exercise in order to optimize your body's ability to bounce back afterward.

Please, don't try to work out harder and cut calories at the same time. Your body will rebel against this and you will likely end up feeling more tired and hate working out. The goal here is to make your body feel great about exercising and be motivated to keep going. Eating some carbs while exercising can help with that. So can making sure that you are eating soon after exercising, so you don't signal your body to go into starvation mode where it burns fewer calories and sabotages your attempts at weight loss. If you want to cut calories, do it in the evening, between dinner and bedtime when you would ordinarily snack. If you feed your body properly, you may well find that you don't feel the munchies then at all.

Sometimes in our colloquial way of talking we say we feel "guilty" about indulging ourselves in a piece of chocolate cake or some other treat. I do this too, but a friend of mine made a comment to me that eating food is not a moral choice and I agree with her. (Ethical vegetarians and vegans may disagree on this.) Still, if you are eating chocolate, you are not a bad person. Eating chocolate or a piece of cheesecake or even a steak doesn't make you evil. It doesn't prove that you lack self-control, either. I think we, as a culture, put far too much emphasis on the link between character and body shape. You cannot judge a book by its cover, or a person by their body.

If you ate a piece of chocolate cake in celebration of a birthday or another occasion, good for you. People need to celebrate. If you need a pick me up, go for it. If you find yourself indulging too often for your own comfort, then maybe you are trying to give yourself something that food isn't actually able to give you. Or maybe you are eating the wrong kind of food hoping it will help you feel full, and it doesn't. Sometimes in America we are so obsessed with measuring calories and vitamins that we eat a processed sports bar when a handful of nuts and a piece of fresh fruit would help us feel better and give us a lot more nutrition.

Most importantly, give yourself a break. Don't beat yourself up over what you eat. Focus on the important things in life. If you are unhappy, figure out what makes you happy. I suspect that most people enjoy the endorphins that are naturally released chemicals in your brain when you do even light exercise. Go outside, walk a little, see the sunset, visit friends. Have a good life, and make exercise and good food part of that good life.

Eating Healthy Tips

Five Healthy Eating Guidelines

1. Avoid Processed Food

   This just means that eating whole fruit (rather than juiced) is better for you. It means eating a tomato is probably better than tomato sauce on a pizza. If you eat crackers, try to look at the ingredients list and get crackers that have fewer ingredients, especially fewer of those you can't pronounce or that look like they are written in Latin or science-ese.

2. Eat More Vegetables and Fruits

   The one thing that I agree with when I talk to people who believe in low-carb diets is that most Americans are not eating enough fruits and vegetables. Try to get in a salad at least once a day. I say this as someone who used to complain that she wasn't a rabbit. Find out what kind of lettuce you like (I prefer either spinach or mixed greens—anything but tasteless iceberg). Then add to the salad things that you will like. If you like dried fruits, keep those on hand so you can always eat a yummy salad. If you like nuts, put on a few (keep away from nuts that have a lot of sugar added). Go for a light oil and vinegar based dressing. Add a little cheese if you like (but not too much).

3. Cut Back on Your Red Meat Consumption

   Not everyone has the commitment to be a vegetarian, and that's fine. But anyone can choose healthier options at home or at a restaurant. Fish instead of red meat is much healthier for you, in part because red meat tends to be much higher in fat, but also because the fat in fish like salmon is a healthier kind of fat.

4. Stay Away From Saturated Fat

This means that butter, cheese, and cream are not your friends. Yes, I admit they are delicious. I love my cheese. It's one of the reasons I could not be a vegan for long. But think of cheese as a condiment. Use it sparingly. If you have pizza, try to keep it to a single piece and don't load up on all those unhealthy, fatty meats on top; try topping it with some mushrooms, spinach and zucchini instead.

5. Try to Expand Your Food Repertoire

Americans tend to eat the same three fruits every day: apples, bananas, oranges. For better health, try a lot of different kinds of fruits. Experiment with mangoes, papayas, and kiwis. If you see a fruit you haven't tried before in the grocery store, like a persimmon or huckleberries, give them a try. Variety is extremely healthy. And as for vegetables, when I became a vegetarian about seven years ago, I realized that I had been limiting myself to onions, potatoes, and carrots for too long. Now we eat turnips and parsnips, okra and eggplant, peppers of all colors, sprouts, and on and on. We live in a country of plenty, so take advantage of it.

10 Foods to Fuel Your Workouts

The more you are pushing your body to perform, the more you need to eat the healthiest snacks to get the most nutrition you can to your body.

1. A handful of nuts (15–20 almonds, for instance) and a piece of fruit (like an apple or a pear)

2. Carrot and celery sticks with a tablespoon peanut butter

3. A handful of raisins or other dried fruit (like apricots) with 1/2 cup of non-fat, plain yogurt (Don't get dried fruit with tons of sugar added like most bananas, papayas, or mangos.)

4. 10–15 olives, green or black, with a cup of soymilk

5. One pickle (if you don't have a sodium-restricted diet) or 1/2 cup of sliced beets with 1/2 cup chickpeas

6. 1 ounce of corn chips and 1/4 cup of healthy, low-fat bean dip

7. 1 piece of wheat toast and 1 cup of bean soup

8. 1/4 cup low-fat hummus and 1 ounce of baked pita chips

9. A banana sliced into 1/2 cup non-fat, plain yogurt

10. 2 ounces of tofu chunks with 1/2 cup of fresh berries

10 Things to Eat (or Drink) While Exercising

1. Gatorade of any flavor or PowerAde—any sports drink that contains sucrose. (Beware of taste fatigue here. If you drink too much of the same flavor, you may stop wanting to take it in, so try to have different flavors around.)

2. Sports gels of a flavor that you like. (Again, beware of taste fatigue.)

3. Sports chews like GU chomps or Clif Shot Blocks.

4. Jelly beans or sports beans (if you feel you need salt).

5. Grapes or bananas (apples and other fruits probably have too much fiber for use while exercising).

6. Pretzels (if you can stand the dry taste in the mouth).

7. Many long distance runners and cyclists eat peanut butter and jelly sandwiches—easy on the PB because you don't want too much protein while exercising, save the protein for after.

8. Gummy bears or cinnamon bears.

9. Pop tarts or cold cereal in a bag. (Be careful it doesn't have too much fiber.)

10. Sports bars that are low in protein and fiber. (Look at labels and judge by what works for you. I can eat Clif bars during cycling, but not during running.)

You can eat too many calories during exercise, and that can cause you to have significant gastric distress. If you walk it off, you will probably be all right in an hour or so. For men, the guidelines are usually three to four hundred calories per hour and for women two to three hundred calories, but this can vary widely and you may have to try out what works best for you. Sometimes you have to practice getting your body to use calories while exercising if you haven't done it before. Don't give up. Your body will figure this out.

Tips For Weight Training

Weight training is a great way to prevent injuries and age-related muscle loss. Now, you don't necessarily have to go to the gym and use machines to do weight lifting. You can do yoga or Pilates. You can get an exersice ball and do exercises while you watch TV. You can do it all without ever once lifting any barbells or dumbbells and using the weight only of your own body. But that said, you should do some weight lifting twice a week for twenty to thirty minutes. Once you get used to it, it really is not that hard. You won't be huffing and puffing like you do during a cardio workout, and if you are really sore the next day, you're doing too much. You should just feel a bit sluggish in the muscles you workout the next day, but not so much that you can't do an easy cardio workout.

Guidelines

Do 3 Sets of 10 Reps for Each Exercise

This means you choose a weight that is easy enough that you can do ten reps with it and still feel like you could do a couple more. I would caution most people to aim for lower than they think especially the first little while. You will be pretty sore the first few weeks. That's perfectly normal. You may not feel pain while working out, so be gentle on yourself. You can always go up for the next set.

Choose 5 to 6 Different Exercises Per Session

This means don't just do one weight lifting exercise and call it done. You can either focus on upper body or lower body or do all of them together. But make sure you aren't doing three exercises that all focus on triceps, either.

Prioritize Major Muscle Groups over Minor Ones

This means do chin-ups or assisted chin-ups or dips over isolated bicep presses. Do chest presses instead of triceps work. Work your hamstrings and quads rather than just your calf muscles. Work out as many muscles at the same time as you can. So pushups, which work almost everything, are superb. Also, almost anything where you are using your own body weight is better than a weight machine isolated exercise because your body is what you use all the time. Lunges, therefore, are better in my mind than leg presses at the gym.

Do Circuit Training

This means that instead of working on one muscle group at a time, resting for a minute, and then doing that same exercise again, I do the whole set of exercises without any rest in between, then start at the beginning again. Take about ten minutes per circuit.

Don't Do the Same Exercises All the Time

Try to change muscle group focus for your two workouts and repeat after one full week. This helps with boredom and recovery at the same time. Change things up as much as possible. I don't want to do lunges every work out for a month.

Do Core/Abdominal Work Every Time

You don't have to do the same sit-ups every time (I do a lot of sit-ups—they're good for you), but there are a ton of exercises that work that area. You can do leg lifts, standing lifts, even chin-ups to work your abs. Sitting on a ball works them. And never *ever* use the abdominal machine at the gym. It's worthless, seriously.

Endnotes

1. "About BMI for Adults," Centers for Disease Control and Prevention, last modified September 13, 2011, http://www.cdc.gov/healthyweight/assessing/bmi/adult_bmi/index.html.

2. Carolyn E. Moore et al. "The Relationship of Exercise and Diet on High-Density Lipoprotein Cholesterol Levels in Women." *Metabolism* 32, no. 2 (1983):189–196.

3. J. Malcolm Arnold et al. "Resting Heart Rate: A Modifiable Prognostic Indicator of Cardiovascular Risk and Outcomes." *The Canadian Journal of Cardiology* 24, Suppl A (2008): 3A–8A.

4. Deborah Kotz, "Stopping Age-Related Muscle Loss." *The Boston Globe*, March 5, 2012, http://www.boston.com/lifestyle/health/articles/2012/03/05/stopping_age_related_muscle_loss/

5. "How Much Physical Activity Do Older Adults Need?" Centers for Disease Control and Prevention, last modified December 1, 2011, http://www.cdc.gov/physicalactivity/everyone/guidelines/olderadults.html.

6. Andrew P. Wroblewski et al. "Chronic Exercise Preserves Lean Muscle Mass in Masters Athletes." The Physician and Sportsmedicine 39, no. 3 (2011):172–178. doi: 10.3810/psm.2011.09.1933.

7. Asker Jeukendrup, Michael Gleeson, *Sport Nutrition* (Champaign, IL:Human Kinetics Publishers, 2010).

8. Douglas Fox, "The Brain May Not Be Fooled by Sugar Substitutes." *Los Angeles Times*, August 31, 2009, http://articles.latimes.com/2009/aug/31/health/he-sweet-brain31.

9. Janice Lloyd, "Protein Pulls Ahead on the Post-Workout Menu," *USA Today*, February 15, 2009, http://usatoday30.usatoday.com/news/health/2009-02-11-protein-recovery_N.htm.

CHAPTER 6

DIFFERENT KIDS: DIFFERENT STROKES

Not Every Kid Is Born to Win, But Everyone Can Succeed

The summer I trained for my first Ironman, my kids began to show some interest in doing something athletic themselves. This wasn't something I had expected, in part because my own childhood had been lacking in athletics, and in part because I had never been the kind of parent who pressed each child to choose a sport. I was happy to pay for lessons or sports, but I wanted to wait until my children told me what they wanted to do. Organized sports had never been my thing, and even if I wanted my kids to be fit, I didn't necessarily think that meant they had to do races or join a team. Our children's fitness regimen included walking to school each day, family outings at the parks, and family hikes in the mountains.

When my oldest daughter, Hope, announced that she wanted to be on the local swim team, I was pleased. We signed Hope up for the "Surfers" at our local pool. This really marked the beginning of family training. I had never really intended to make triathlon into a family activity. It was a very personal experience, but I loved it so much that I think the kids wanted to experience it in their own way. At first, the kids did their own thing, and I did mine.

Some days I would take Hope to swim team in the mornings and do my own workouts as she did hers. Her favorite coach was Royal, a young lifeguard who had helped time me for competitive swims. He was always cheerful and kind, never yelling at swimmers, and always offering help.

That first year, Hope was swimming nearly every day for an hour or more. She seemed like a little fish, naturally suited to the water. I'd put all the kids through the series of Red Cross swim classes levels one through six that are offered locally just about anywhere. Hope had completed the last level the summer before, qualifying her to join the team. She rapidly moved up from the first group of swimmers and actually regretted it, since it meant she was no longer with Royal. Now Hope was ready to go to swim meets with the team.

Soon Sage (then ten) and Faith (then six) asked if they could join the team. It was easier for them to imagine joining a swim team if they knew that Hope would be there in the same lane with them, showing them every step.

Neither Sage nor Faith was ready to do competitions that first year, but I remember driving for an hour so Hope could do an invitational swim meet at a big outdoor pool. She was sick with fear of what would happen when she got up on the blocks. There are so many things to worry about when you are swimming. If you dive in before the gun goes off, everyone must start all over again. If you do it twice, you'll be disqualified. Being disqualified or DQ'd was one of Hope's greatest fears. It can happen in a dozen different ways. The judges watch you as you swim and can DQ you if you aren't doing the right stroke, or aren't doing it properly the whole race.

In the end, Hope did just fine. She ended up taking fifth place in her age group for one of the events and we got her a little trophy for it. I took the kids down and we all got to see her do her best, and while it was difficult for me, I was glad that it became a family event. She loved swimming and would always say she would rather swim a mile than run it, even if swimming took four times as long.

Hope continued swimming into her high school years. She never went to State. She didn't win a lot of races. But she was always an asset to the team. She ended up specializing in some of the hardest racing events and was willing to swim races that other swimmers shied away from. Her standard races were the five hundred-yard freestyle, which is the longest race, and the 200 Individual Medley where you do fifty yards of each stroke: back, breast, fly, and free. Other kids tended to get DQ'd in the two hundred IM because you can make a mistake in each stroke, but Hope has beautiful technique in all the strokes. So, even if she wasn't as fast, she'd make points for the team.

One of the best moments for Matt and me as parents was the end-of-season dinner where all the families got together to see their kids receive awards. Hope didn't get a letter every year, but she did get an award every year for being the nicest or the "smilingest" kid on the team. I only had to mention Hope's name to the other swimmers or parents and they instantly knew who she was. Sometimes they would come and ask me why Hope was always so happy. I don't know why. That's the way she is. No matter how hard she is working out, she still has a smile on her face. She doesn't get that from me, but it's a great thing to have in the family.

Her senior year, Hope decided not to go back to the swim team. That was a little disappointing, but she ended up feeling like she needed to devote more time to her academics. She didn't give up an athletic lifestyle, however. She trained for Olympic triathlons, a half marathon, and a half Ironman with us as a family over the next year before she headed off to college, so I consider that a success.

Find What Motivates Your Child

In 2007, we moved to a different pool and the younger kids changed to a new city team with all new coaches. Sage and Faith continued to swim for the team, but they struggled. They didn't have the same temperament as Hope and they didn't deal well with the pressure the coaches put on them to get ready to compete. Everything about the new team seemed to focus on competition, and even though I often give adults the advice that if they want to get in better shape, they should sign up for a race and train for it, this isn't true for everyone. Some people are affected negatively by the stress and pressure of competition and it makes them want to give up. These people need more internal goals and more individual-based goals to keep them motivated.

This may ring true to you if you have a more internally motivated child or are more internally motivated yourself. In the first swim meet Sage and Faith went to, Sage was terrified of being on the starting blocks. She started one race, nearly falling into the water and drowning while everyone else was swimming. Finally, she got out dead last, shivering and upset with tears dripping down her cheeks. Her face turned red and she put her arms around her legs and rocked back and forth in distress. When it was time for her to get up on the blocks for the next race, she just refused to do it.

Matt and I were up in the stands watching her talk to the coach, and the coach glanced up at us in a plea to come down and talk to her. I trooped down to the pool area and did my best to coax her. But nothing I promised Sage as a reward or any of her coach's pleading on behalf of the team had any effect on her. Sage is like that, very stubborn. In some ways, it's a good thing (I tell myself, anyway). If my kids won't listen to me when I try to talk them into something, that means they won't listen to other people, like stupid friends, who try to talk them into doing something dangerous. Right?

Finally, I told the coach that Sage needed a break. I brought her up to the stands with me. I got her some food and she felt a little better, but she would not enter another race. I felt embarrassed that she had acted that way, but I tried to do what was best for Sage. She enjoyed swimming, but she needed me to go to bat for her with the coaches. I told them she wanted to still be on the team, to go to workouts every day, but not the competitions. Sadly, the coaches didn't react well to this and insisted that the only way to improve was to compete. They let her remain on the younger, non-competitive team, but after a few months, the negative attitude of the coaches was clear. They didn't want her on the team. They didn't value her. So we ended up finding our own strategies to motivate Sage in a different way.

Sage seemed to like running more than swimming, and we signed her up for some smaller races. She especially seemed to dislike team sports, and, after some bad falls, she doesn't like bike riding much at all. Nonetheless, Sage is competitive in her own way. Sage has known since she was very young that she wanted to sing professionally. In some ways she comes alive on stage in a way that she isn't alive anywhere else. She received an honorable mention in the Utah State Fair at age eleven, five years before she was technically old enough to compete. She has written and produced her own album of original songs, and she has performed in multiple school plays and music competitions. In 2013, she was accepted to Berklee School of Music in Boston, one of the top music colleges in the country, with a good scholarship. Her love is the stage rather than the pavement or pool, but that doesn't mean she never wants to do athletic things.

Sage hasn't done many triathlon competitions with us as a family, but in 2012, she agreed to do the Salt Lake Half Marathon with the rest of the family (minus Zach, then age ten). Following my Christmas present training plan, Sage was diligent in preparing for the running leg of the triathlon. I ran a couple of long runs with her, and she ended up doing much better than we expected, finishing in 2:30. She has since done two more half marathons, progressively improving to 2:13 and then 2:03.

As you work to find what works for you and your family, keep in mind that people need different things to improve. Some people need to find what they truly love, like Sage's singing. Some need competition and medals. Others need only an encouraging word. Find what motivates your kids and find what motivates you. Then you will be on your way.

Beginning Swimming Tips

It can be difficult to learn how to swim as an adult, especially if you have focused mainly on running or biking in the past. The rules are very different. Whereas running and biking are all about your heart and aerobic capacity, swimming is all about your technique.

Getting Started

True Beginners

Of course, if you are a beginner and have never learned how to swim before (like my mother-in-law who faced down her fear of water at the age of fifty-five), you will need to either take an adult swim class at a local pool, or, if that embarrasses you, hire one of the swim teachers at a local pool for private lessons. These are usually priced very reasonably. Group lessons cost about ten dollars a lesson for one half hour. A private lesson shouldn't cost more than twenty to thirty dollars for a half hour. Sometimes private lessons end up being a lot less expensive in the long run because you can progress faster with individual attention.

Moving to the Next Level

If you know the basics of swimming, and can go from one end of the pool to the other without drowning, you are probably ready to move on to the next step. It is time to join an adult team or to simply go work out at the pool on a regular basis. You can watch other swimmers, either on top of the water, or with goggles underneath to observe proper swim technique. A coach can tell you what you're doing and how to improve, or you can have a friend come and make a video of you swimming. Analyze it and compare with videos of professional swimmers online. Another source for studying technique is YouTube. On YouTube if you type in "total immersion" there are a lot of videos like this one: http://www.youtube.com/watch?v=V3UqGYhbNN4&feature=related

"Total Immersion" is a swimming style for triathletes designed to make freestyle swimming easier and to help you save energy for the run and the bike. It is also just plain good swimming.

Master Swimming

If you are looking for a great website with videos, drawings, and articles that offer advice on swimming, go to usms.org. USMS or United States Master Swimming is the gateway to competitive swimming as an adult. They host many races locally, and others you can do "postally" (i.e. at your own pool and send the results in). Some of the articles, and most of the races, on the site are only available if you are a member. Membership in the USMS costs about fifty dollars a year. I think it is worth it, even if you don't do a lot of swim racing. If you sign up in November of one year, you can get membership to the end of that year and for the entire next year all bundled into one price.

Racing

If you are worried about going to Master Swim races as a beginner, let me assure that there are all kinds of swimmers. You are asked your estimated swim time and will be put in a proper group of like swimmers for your heat. There will be other beginners, and also people who have had cancer or brain injuries returning to activity. It can be really inspiring. You will see everything from people who are in their eighties and nineties to those who are trying to set world records for Masters. Don't worry about looking slim and perfect in a suit either. I once got up on the blocks next to a guy with quite a bit of a gut. He was in his fifties and was coming back after being a star swimmer in high school. I was sure I would beat him, but he blew right past me. In the water, a little extra fat can actually be an advantage in buoyancy. You will see all body types.

The Basics of Proper Technique

When I watch adults who are getting back into swimming, I notice first of all that they are uncomfortable and often desperate for breath. As you begin to get yourself into swimming shape, you should float in the water, and feel comfortable. If you don't feel comfortable, you just need to spend more time in the pool, and don't worry at first about your speed. *A basic rule of thumb is that when you can swim a lap (fifty yards) in about a minute, you are ready to work on speed. Before that, focus on technique.* Here are some simple points of technique anyone can work on.

Relax

Remember that your body is naturally buoyant and relax. You're not going to start to drown if you stop stroking. Remember this as you do all of the drills.

Even Stroke

You need to make sure that your stroke is even. A pool helps you with lines at the bottom, but if you tend to pull on either side, this will be exaggerated in an open water triathlon swim. See drills 1 and 2.

Breathe on Both Sides

Feel free to breathe every stroke if you need to, but it's useful to know how to breathe on both sides to even things out. Many people who breathe on only one side end up having imbalances that can lead to later fatigue or injury. See drill 2.

Rotate Your Whole Body

As you stroke, your whole body turns from side to side. This means that your hips and your torso and your shoulders should all point to the bottom of the pool mid-stroke, then go horizontal and turn again when you stroke to the other side. Think of your whole upper body and hips following your arm down into the water. See drill 3.

Pure Glide

You should have a part of your stroke that is pure glide, where you aren't working at all. See drills 4 and 5.

Bend Your Elbows

When you pull up your arms, your elbow should be bent so you do not use extra energy swinging your arm in a windmill stroke. See drill 6.

Complete Your Stroke

Make sure that you complete every stroke from the moment you touch the water above your head to when the hand comes out of the water at about hip level. This will help you greatly to relax in the water and use less energy. See drill 7.

Straight Reach

You should also try to reach out directly in front of your shoulders, so your arm is straight, not crossing over in front of your head. Crossing over above your head is wasted energy and will unbalance you. See drill 8.

Hands Slightly Open

Sometimes beginning swimmers spend a lot of energy trying to keep their fingers held tightly together in a "scoop." This is unnecessary and isn't proper swim technique. Hold your fingers slightly curved and with a little bit of space between them. Don't think too much about the hand. Your swim stroke is really more about your whole body. See drills 1 and 9.

Work Your Legs

Remember that you are not simply using your arms to scoop water away from your body. Your legs must work as well. Focus on a smooth, rhythmic, short kick up and down. See drill 10.

Body Position

Keep your body position high in the water. Most of your back and shoulder will be out of the water as you recover from side to side. See drill 11.

Make a Movie

Ask someone to video you for a few minutes, so you can see what you are doing. You will be able to spot some of your weak areas just by looking at the video. You can also ask a lifeguard at the pool to give you tips. Then you can focus on drills that will help to deal with your weaknesses.

You may even see people doing a "flip turn" at the end of the wall like swimmers do in the Olympics. This is a useful skill for pool races, but not much use in triathlon, so I won't address it here.

Drills

Once you are swimming well and comfortable with the crawl/free-style, you should start some drills to improve your skills and get you moving through the water a little faster. Here are some drills I recommend. I do ten laps, one lap of each drill I need to focus on, at the beginning of every workout. This helps set the proper technique into my head and into my muscle memory. It's also a great warm up.

Some swimmers take paper to the pool with a workout written on it. Be aware that your paper will get wet and soggy and may become unreadable toward the end of the workout. You could also memorize your workout or laminate it.

One Arm Drill

Swim with your left arm only on the way out, your right arm only on the way back. This helps even out your stroke.

Breathing Drill

Breathe every third stroke, every fifth, every seventh, every ninth. Your lung capacity will increase and alternating your breathing from left to right will become more natural.

Rolling Drill

With each stroke, take plenty of time and make sure you roll completely from right to left, so that your shoulders are perpendicular to the surface of the water with each stroke.

Golf Drill

Swim one length of the pool while counting strokes. Now swim the length again trying to decrease the number of stokes you need to cross the pool. A really good swimmer can get away with three to four strokes for a whole pool length. Beginners need more like fifteen to twenty. Keep track of your progress. This forces you to glide more.

Catch Up Drill:

Don't take the next stroke until the other arm touches your fingers above your head. Again, this teaches you to glide and relax.

High Elbow Recovery

Instead of lifting your arm out of the water hand first and flinging the whole arm windmill style out of the water, take the elbow out first and hold the rest of your arm underneath, kind of like a chicken, and push the hand forward through the water. Do not let your hand come completely out of the water. This ensures that you don't bring your hand up too far and are using the most efficient stroke possible.

Final Push

Focus on the last part of your stroke. Finish the final part of the stroke from chest level to hip level. You need to push down hard to get every last bit of propulsion from this stroke. If you pull your arm out of the water too early you will cheat yourself of this power.

Shoulder Width Entry Point

Focus on the front part of your stroke and make sure you aren't crossing over your head with either arm. Your hand should hit the water directly in front of your shoulder.

Fist Drill

Swim with your fists closed. This helps you think about other parts of your arm that propel you forward, not just your hand.

Side Kick Drill

Use a kickboard and roll from side to side, counting four strokes on one side and then four on the other. A lot of standard kickboard drills that have you simply kick while horizontal in the water don't really mimic the way that you will be kicking as your body turns from side to side.

Catch Drill

This drill is named for the first part of the stroke when your hand enters the water and "catches" it. Focus on the front part of the stroke and really dig into it, punching hard into the water. This will also help your body position because it forces you to turn to the side and keep your head high.

Note: many of these drills exaggerate normal swim stroke in order to make a point. Obviously, there is no need for your hands to touch above your head as in drill 4 or for you to drag your hand through the water through the entire recovery portion of the stroke.

Swimming Gear

The most important thing is to get into the water and swim. You can manage with just a swim suit and even no goggles, though I recommend getting goggles as soon as you can to encourage keeping your head in the water. Other equipment is nice, but don't feel like you have to spend a lot of money to go swimming. Start with the basics and then acquire other equipment one piece at a time. Also, many swimming pools will have this equipment on hand to borrow. I have listed the swimming gear from most important to least important, but feel free to decide what you think would be most useful for you.

Swimsuit

As for swimsuits, please do not buy a Lycra suit from your typical department store. Lycra suits disintegrate quickly with regular use. They are meant to make you look good while you lounge around a pool, and are not for actual swimming. The best place to buy suits online is www.swimoutlet.com. Look for polyester suits; they will last for years. There are men's suits that are available in the same fabric called Jammers. They are long enough to be modest and comfortable. Mini Speedo suits are no longer the standard that they were when I was in high school. Girls and boys can buy suits at www.swimoutlet.com, as well. They stock in all sizes and styles and there are lots of colors to choose from. I like a plain black suit, but my fashion-conscious daughter, Sage, is always looking for one that is more stylish.

Goggles

Get a good pair of goggles—don't get them at the grocery store. You are not going to be able to swim more than a length of the pool in crappy goggles. You will pay between fifteen to twenty dollars for a good pair of goggles. I recommend Speedo Hydrospex, which are the only kind of goggles I ever buy. However, I recently had a friend show me why they were not the right pair for her. She has a bigger nose than I do and they simply don't work for her face shape. She prefers Speedo Vanquisher. You may have to buy several different pairs before you figure out which one is right for you. I replace goggles every three or four months. When they start going foggy, it's time for a new pair. You can try putting anti-fog spray on, but I haven't found it particularly useful. Also, if you start having pain around your eyes after wearing the goggles for more than thirty minutes, that is normal. You'll have to get used to the feeling or simply rest and take them off for a few minutes then put them back on. Your goggle break is a good time to do kickboard work.

Swim Cap

For women, you will want to have a swim cap unless you have very short hair. You can get cheap latex ones for a couple of dollars, but don't. Buy the silicone ones that cost about ten dollars and last forever. I bought one at the Ironman in 2004 and it lasted for six years. I swim a lot, so that says something. The silicone caps don't rip like the latex ones do and they don't pull on your hair as badly either. They are also easier to get on and off. Lycra caps are more comfortable than the other kinds, but last about three swims before they wear out. You know you need to replace your silicone cap when it starts to get discolored or has spots of dark mold on it.

Fins/Flippers

You can do some easier swimming using fins. I think swimming with fins mimics swimming with a wetsuit fairly well since wetsuits help you become more buoyant and use less energy staying up in the water. When you wear a wetsuit you actually do not need to kick as hard, so it feels similar to wearing fins. Fins can also help make it easier to swim for beginners, so you can spend more time in the pool, and more time in the pool means better swimming. But don't wear fins for more than a quarter of your practice laps or time or you can become too dependent on them. You can buy them in any online swim store or at your local sports store. I recommend getting ones that are shorter. "Zoomers" brand are my favorite.

Kickboard

Using a kick board can encourage you to get in more time in the water and to use proper kicking technique while swimming, which is with your feet stretched out, not perpendicular to your legs. Most swimming pools have them on hand. If not, you can buy your own for about ten dollars and take it with you. If you struggle with getting enough breath, use a kickboard on alternating laps, then you can get more distance in and still not feel like you're going hypoxic. If you want to use a kickboard, hold it under your chest; don't hold it stretched out in front of you.

Paddles

Paddles (which look like over-sized hand-shaped pieces of plastic with holes) increase water resistance, working your arms and shoulders like a mini weight lifting workout in the pool. Some people, especially women, need to build up significant upper body strength before they can really slice through the water. That doesn't happen overnight. As with fins, be careful not to use them for more than a quarter of your total workout laps or time. If you use them too much, you can end up with overuse injuries on your shoulders. Be aware of your body, if you feel any pain in your shoulders, lay off the paddles for a while. Don't use them for any stroke other than freestyle. When you use them, really push hard from the top of your stroke to the bottom. Rest a lot in between each lap.

Tether

If you are a business person and spend some time out of town at hotels, you know that hotel pools are designed more for playing around than for exercise. You can easily convert a hotel pool into a swim treadmill with a tether from an online swim seller. These tethers cost about twenty dollars and are not much more than stretchy ropes. You tie them around your waist and then to a pool ladder. Then you swim as normal and the tether holds you in place. Matt hates these, and eagerly gave me his after using it only once. The normal movement of his body through the water didn't happen with a tether. He found it frustrating. I used it once and got kind of hooked. It's a great way to add twenty minutes in the pool when I'm at a writing conference. At a hotel, twenty minutes in the pool is great for winding down after a long day. If you hate treadmills and stationary bikes, it may not be for you. Otherwise, you may love it.

Underwater MP3 players

I do not have one of these, but I want to get one. They are expensive, but one of my friends swears by hers. She says that the rhythm of music in the water motivates her to keep going when otherwise she might give up and stop after a few laps. You wear earpieces under goggles and swim cap and then clip the player onto your cap. It's a little extra weight and I imagine it takes getting used to. The only caution I have about this is to be extra aware of other people in your swim lane. If you're digging your tunes, you may not be listening to the normal sounds around you and may end up interfering with other swimmers.

Shampoo

One thing that many women and some men swear by is shampoo for swimmers. I have met swimmers who had Incredible Hulk style green hair after spending hours a day in the pool. I swim two or three times a week and I don't blow dry my hair or use a curling iron on it. My hair stylist tells me I have supremely healthy hair, so I don't worry about special shampoo. If the smell of chlorine really bothers you, it might be worth it for you to get special shampoo or shower gel. If you have blonde hair that shows a color change from swimming, definitely get it. Use it every time you swim.

Swim Bag

There are many expensive swim bags you can buy, or you can just throw everything in a backpack, as long as you air it out. I have a special swim bag made of a material that lets water drip out easily. It has a zip pocket for my soap, shampoo and razor and another pocket for my gym membership card, a comb, and some cash for emergencies. There is a large section for everything else. I also use a small mesh bag that I keep my goggles, fins, cap, and paddles in. This makes my poolside gear easy to grab and quick to dry when I put it away. It also helps to wrap your wet swimsuit in a towel so it doesn't drip in your bag.

Wetsuit

If you are going to do an open water swim, you will probably need a wetsuit. You can buy a wetsuit at many specialty swim shops and sometimes at bike or running stores that cater to triathletes. These are not the same kinds of wetsuits you would buy for waterskiing. I've seen people try to use those, and while they keep you warm, they also drag you down and make you much slower. TYR, Zoot, and BlueSeventy all make great triathlon wetsuits. Be aware that a good wetsuit will cost at least two hundred dollars, maybe a little less if you find it on sale. Look for sizing recommendations based on your height and weight and sex. Most wetsuits have a zipper up the back and are very difficult to get on, especially the first time. They are very tight-fitting and are made of state of the art materials to keep you buoyant. With a wetsuit on, it is almost impossible for you to sink in an open water swim. They are uncomfortable and hot, so don't put it on until about twenty minutes before the race starts.

BodyGlide

You'll need something like Body Glide to rub all over your calves, ankles, arms, wrists, and neck to keep the suit from chafing your body and giving you sores for days afterward. Some people use Pam; don't use vaseline as it can damage your wetsuit. It also helps the suit slip off when the race is done. Some races will have wetsuit strippers to help you out of your suit, but for most, you will spend a minute or so getting out of it.

Rules for Pool Swimming

I have been swimming laps since I was fourteen, which is almost thirty years now. When I started on the swim team, I had no idea what I was doing. We'd had a swimming pool in the backyard when I was a kid, but I'd never had formal swimming lessons until a month before the swim team started. I only knew vaguely that there was more than one swimming stroke, or that you were supposed to dive into a pool in a particular way. I didn't know at all how to breathe while swimming, how to do a flip turn or how to circle swim. The rules for swim team swimming are really useful to learn, even if you're not on a swim team because they are the same you follow for lap swimming as you train. Here are the basics.

Circle Swim

If there are more than two people swimming in a lane, you must circle swim. This is done by swimming up the right hand side of the lane, as if you are driving a car, then flipping or turning at the end, and continuing to swim on the right hand side.

Passing

If you swim slowly, expect that the other swimmers in the pool will need to pass you. Try to be aware of where they are and stop at the side of the pool for them to pass you if they are coming close. If they are expert swimmers, they will not be willing to wait for a turn and will touch your foot when they need to pass. Your job then is not to stop (although you can if you choose to), but to move as far to the right as you can. Again, as in driving a car, the center section of the lane now becomes the passing section and the faster swimmer will move around you as quickly as possible. If this happens often, it can be annoying, but it's just the way that it is. You can try to find a lane that is designated "slow" swimming. Still, remember, there is no need to apologize about being slow. You have as much right to be in the swim lane as anyone.

Side-to-Side Swimming

If there are only two people in a lane, or if you are swimming alone, I recommend side to side swimming. This allows two swimmers of varying abilities to swim in the same lane without ever bothering each other. If you are swimming on the left side of the lane, you flip and keep on that side, though now it will be on the right. Just stay on your side, and you won't ever cross paths with the other swimmer.

Don't Hog a Lane

It is considered rude if you are in a lane by yourself and decide to swim right down the middle on the black line. I may just get in the lane with you anyway and start swimming to one side and expect you to move over politely. There is no reason that one person should be allowed to take a lane all by him or herself.

Ask For Advice

If you are feeling chatty at the swimming pool during a break, feel free to talk to other swimmers who are resting at the side of the pool. I generally find that other swimmers are happy to give advice about swimming, or gear, or weight loss, or whatever you are interested in. You'd be surprised at how many swimmers would love to give you advice about your stroke. My husband is always itching to tell people how to be more efficient swimmers. It's like listening to someone play a violin off-key to him. It just bothers him to see weird strokes. So, if you see someone better than you taking a break, ask for advice.

Swimming in Open Water

When I did my first race, I had no experience doing an open water swim. I was terrified the first ten minutes and was sure I was going to die. But I eventually got into a rhythm and figured out how to keep going.

Getting a Feel for Open Water

While there is nothing quite like a mass swim start, you can at least get an idea of how it feels to swim in open water where you often cannot see anything in front of you by going to a nearby lake or reservoir and putting on a wetsuit. Start by walking a few feet out from the shore. When the water is about knee height, you can lean forward and start swimming. It will feel weird and a little cold as the water seeps into the wetsuit. This is normal. Don't panic. Just keep swimming. A wetsuit can also restrict your shoulder movements a little and make it more difficult to do a proper high elbow recovery. Just do your best. If you really dislike a full wetsuit, you can buy a sleeveless one that will restrict your movement less.

Note: Don't try to wear a wetsuit in a pool. Pool water temperature is usually kept at above eighty, which is the danger zone for wetsuits. Wetsuits are made to keep you warm, and if water temperature is above eighty, wetsuits are not allowed in triathlon races. This is for safety, because you can get overheated and become very ill.

Sighting

In an open water swim training exercise, you won't have buoys marked out to show you exactly where to go or to indicate how far you've gone. I often will try to "sight" some of the buoys that are set out to prevent boats from coming into the swim areas. Then I swim just the shore side of those buoys in a long line. I swim back and forth along the same buoy line so I don't get lost in a new area. Swimming alongside the buoys is good practice for trying to "sight" the buoys for a triathlon.

Counting Strokes

I count strokes to give me some idea of how far I have gone, one for each separate arm motion. Usually about one stroke equals a meter. Count to a hundred and then start over again. If you swim absolutely straight, 3800 meters is a full Ironman triathlon, 1900 meters a half Ironman, 1500 meters an Olympic distance, and 750 meters a sprint. You can also check your watch to see how long you have been in the water to get an idea of how far you have to go.

Sun in Your Eyes

Another challenge is swimming as the sun is rising. It can be hard to see anything around you with the sun shining off your goggles. This is one reason why some people will buy colored lenses for their goggles. I think it's difficult no matter what color the lenses are. For me, it works best to look for someone else who is swimming confidently and follow them. Swimming toward either a sunset or a sunrise in training is good practice.

Mass Starts and Waves

If you want to learn how to deal with waves and a mass swim start without actually doing a race, my best suggestion is to find a master's team with other triathletes. You can all swim in the same lane and ask other swimmers to use kickboards to create "waves" that you have to navigate. A group of ten people in the same lane will feel like the cramped quarters of a race start. Your goggles may get knocked off; that's good practice. It happens in races. Sometimes racers will put on goggles under their caps (or on top of a second cap below the required race one) to try to protect them from getting completely lost in the water. I've had to swim parts of races without goggles. You survive. Just keep your head down and move forward.

Dealing with Phobias

It can be difficult to psych yourself up for an open water swim if you are someone who is hyperconscious of germs and creatures. My oldest daughter Hope is always talking about fear of sharks in a lake, which is silly, but I think what she means is that she is afraid of other living things touching her in the water. It does happen sometimes, but more often the fish swim away, especially if a race is going on and there are a lot of other people in the water. More often, if you feel something touching you in the water, it is a branch or some seaweed. It may feel weird, but don't let it ruin your swim. You can brush it off and keep going. Try not to swallow too much dirty water. Sometimes people do get ill from open water swimming, but it has never happened to me. You are going to be doing so much good for your immune system by exercise that you'll win out in the end.

Your First Open Water Race

Doing your first open water swim race is a difficult undertaking. I recommend doing a pool triathlon first, which will have a shorter swim and will obviously be more comfortable, since you are used to swimming in a pool. But if you've been swimming a year or so in the pool, it's time to try a few open water swims in a local reservoir or lake. Then you may be ready to do an open water triathlon. It's normal to be a little nervous.

Just a rule of thumb: any yard swim is ten percent shorter than the same distance in meters. So if you're doing a 400-meter pool swim in a race, the approximate amount of yards to swim in preparation is 440, or 450 to round off. If you are doing an open water swim, be more generous than ten percent going from yards to meters because you may not swim in a straight line. I try to get in one open water swim a week during the summer to prepare for races.

How Far Should I Go? An Ironman swim is 2.4 miles or 3800 meters normally, although waves can make it seem A LOT longer. Really good swimmers can do this in under an hour in good conditions. I swim about 1:10-1:15 in smooth water. I don't recommend an Ironman swim for beginners AT ALL. You'll want to have been swimming for three to four years before you feel confident enough for that. It is also a good idea to have a buddy with you for any open water swimming. A half Ironman is obviously half of the Ironman, or 1.2 miles. An Olympic swim normally has a 1500 meter swim (or just about a mile which is seventy-two laps in a typical 25-yard pool). I can swim an Olympic distance race now in under twenty-five minutes. Pro men can swim it in under twenty minutes. Under thirty minutes for a first open water swim would be fantastic. Aim for coming in under forty minutes to be realistic.

When you are ready to try your first open water swim, I recommend beginning with an Olympic distance race rather than the shorter sprint, so long as you have worked up the endurance for it during your pool swimming. If you can swim 2000 yards in the pool in forty minutes without trouble, you can do an Olympic distance open water swim (1500 meters), even allowing for a few mistakes in sighting. Almost all triathlon races run a sprint and an Olympic distance on the same day. The sprint starts a little later, but the Olympic will almost always have a much smaller group of people starting at the same time. This can help decrease some of your anxieties about swimming because you won't get knocked around as much, but there will still be other swimmers to follow and help keep you on course.

Having a Successful Race

Here are a few tips to make sure that your first open water swim race isn't terrifying.

Try Out the Race Venue

The best way to deal with nerves about a first race is to go to the race venue and see what the water looks like. You can also see what the transition to the bike is like. Most races will allow you to go the night before at no charge. You can often pick up your race number and T-shirt, then get in the water in your wetsuit and swim around. The race buoys won't be up yet, but it will still be a great way to set youself at ease.

Sleeping

You may have trouble sleeping the night before a race. This is perfectly normal. I think about it as my body revving up for the demands of the race and getting excited for the start time. Do try to sleep as much as you can the week before the race and don't do any hard workouts that week. Most athletes get less than five hours of sleep the night before a race.

Eating Properly

I'm not one for "carb loading" the night before a race, where you go and eat yourself sick on pasta. I do try to eat seventy-five percent carbs and only ten percent fat with ten percent to fifteen percent protein the week before a race. You want to be topping up your body's muscle glycogen stores so that you are at your maximum before the race starts. Three hundred to five hundred grams of carbs per day (depending on your body weight) should do this nicely. The night before a race, don't eat a lot more than you normally would, but don't restrict yourself either. It's a good idea to eat something that you know goes down well. People who race a lot are often a little superstitious about this and will eat the same dinner from the same restaurant before every race. You don't need to go to this extreme, but you do need to avoid new restaurants. I recommend against buffets as well because of the risk of food-borne illness, strange foods, and some personal bad experiences.

It's OK to Wait

If you are doing your first race and are not confident about the swim, you do not have to participate in the mass start. Get in the water with the other swimmers, but don't feel that you have to toe the line with them. When the gun goes off, stay where you are. After about thirty seconds, begin your swim. You will be free of a lot of the craziness. Also, if you stay just a little to the right of everyone else, and go the long way around the buoys, you'll be less likely to have to deal with jostling.

Sight Often

In a pool, you can see the line on the bottom whenever you need to. You have lane lines to help you keep going straight. Often, you will have no idea that your stroke is a little off center until you do an open water swim. Then tiny flaws can be magnified because of the distance. You need to lift your head out of the water a little more when you sight than you ordinarily would just for breathing. Keep track of where the shoreline is, and where the giant orange buoys are. If there are other features you can see, like mountains or a dock with boats along it, look for those to stay on course. If you are confused, stop and figure out where you are, and then go again. For a first time open water swim, you may need to sight every ten strokes. Don't go too many strokes or you will end up swimming a lot of extra meters.

Lifeguards Are There to Help

Be aware that there are kayaks and certified lifeguards in the water at all times around you. The brightly colored swim cap that you will get with your race number in your packet is not just for fun. You are required to wear it for safety reasons. It is to help you stand out in the water. The lifeguards are looking for those caps. With a wetsuit on, it's extremely unlikely that you will drown, but the lifeguards are there to see if anyone goes under or is struggling. They WILL get you out of the water. They do it all the time.

The "Progress" Rule

You can go over to one of the kayaks and simply hang on for a few minutes if you need to. This will not disqualify you. You are only out of the race if you get into the kayak or try to use it to make "progress" through the race course.

Any Stroke Works

If you ever feel like you are short of breath, try doing a stroke that is easier to breathe on. You can flip over onto your back and swim that way, or do breaststroke for as long as you need to. Just make sure you are not in the way of anyone who is trying to swim faster. Stay a little wide of the straight line of the race.

Focus on Finishing

Your first race should be a race to complete, not to compete. Don't try to push yourself to the point of exhaustion the first time out. Since you haven't done this before, you don't know what it feels like every step of the way. You don't know how tired you will be at the end of each discipline. It's better to feel great at the end of the run and sprint the last mile than to end up walking or even worse, having to pull out of the race. I cannot tell you how many times I have seen people who were a lot more fit than I was, puking at the side of the road at races because they started too fast. Take it easy. Like the tortoise, keep moving steadily along, you want to finish the race.

Final Tip: Relax!

I hope this is helpful and makes it a little less scary to get swimming. It's often true that the best thing you can do for your swimming is simply to relax and let your natural buoyancy take over. The more you fight the water, the harder you have to work. You don't need to do super hard swim workouts in order to complete a swim good enough for a triathlon. Go a couple times a week for twenty to thirty minutes. Focus on technique and just get some yards in. Especially for beginners, swimming is not the place for you to do intervals or tempo training. If you do it right, the swim can be the most relaxing part of the race—a warm up to the rest of the day.

CHAPTER 7

WHEN YOU OR YOUR KIDS MAKE MISTAKES

The Definition of Family: A wonderful organization in which things never turn out the way you expect.

One year I wanted to go down to a race for Thanksgiving Day. I had great dreams for this race. I wanted to finish the four-mile race in under 26:00, which was 6:30 per mile. I suppose theoretically I might be able to do that, if I had the perfect day and trained and tapered for it just so. Unfortunately, I spent the day before on my feet in the kitchen, baking pies for the family get together. You know how it goes. You start making a couple of pies and then it gets out of control because you want to make sure everyone has their very favorite pie. I think I must have made a dozen pies.

After all that baking, I was so anxious about my race that I couldn't get to sleep until late. Then we had to get up early to drive down to the race venue with all the kids and the pies in our big green twelve passenger Dodge Ram van, which we affectionately call Hulk. I put the pies on the floor of the van in cardboard boxes to protect them. I reminded the kids several times during the hour long trip that the pies were under their seats and that they might shift during travel. So be careful about the pies.

When we stopped the car, the first thing I said to the kids was, "Look down before you step. Don't step on the pies." I'm sure anyone can guess what happened. Kids are kids, and Sage stepped in two of the pies. Then Sam stepped in two more. Their first reaction wasn't embarrassment at doing exactly what I had told them not to do. It was to complain because the pies had gotten all over their shoes and made them messy.

I mourned over the dead pies I had spent so long working on the day before. Then we found Matt's sister, Rachel, whom we'd asked to come watch the kids while we raced. We waved her over to the car. She came into it and we told her about being careful about the pies (and also, I shoved them back under the seats in hopes they would stay there permanently).

Matt and I went off to get our race numbers put on. We checked back at the car before the race started, and then we headed to the starting line. It is cold in November, of course, and just about at the limit of my endurance for doing a race outside. I wore a long-sleeved shirt, hat and gloves, long pants, and double socks. Matt hates the cold even more than I do, and the worst part was waiting for the start. When the gun finally went off, I pushed as hard as I could, but didn't come anywhere near my goal time. I think I was just under 30:00 for the four miles.

I got back to the car, only to find out that Sage (nine years old at the time) was missing. It was not a good moment. I was too exhausted to deal with things rationally. Sage had told Rachel desperately needed to go to the bathroom and Rachel had been forced to decide between taking Sage to the bathroom or staying with the other kids, three of whom were younger than Sage. She stayed in the car with the younger kids, and Sage got lost on the way back to the car by herself.

We did find Sage about thirty minutes later, crying with some strangers. We got her to do the kids' race, which was a couple hundred yards. I think we tried to get the other kids to run as well, but this was before we had done any track training, and they just refused. We picked up some prizes (including a free pumpkin pie), then loaded everyone back in the car and headed over to Thanksgiving dinner. There were still plenty of pies, and it was a good reminder to me that at Harrison family dinners, there is never a shortage of food.

Every race we do, there is something small that goes wrong. I no longer wish not to forget something. I just hope that what I forget is something that doesn't matter too much. And when you have the whole family racing, things just get more complicated. The chances of something going wrong hover at about 99.9 percent. That's the way it is with a family. People get lost, and you have to find them. Someone misses the race start, and you have to go on without them. We don't expect the kids to be perfect any more than we expect ourselves to be perfect. Being a family means that you love each other even when life does not go perfectly. Races aren't really any different. They just add a little more spice to the problems you already know how to deal with.

How to "Redo" a Race

Another year at the same Thanksgiving Day race, we had talked two of the kids into running with us. It's a double loop course and we explained it to Sam and Hope, but apparently, Sam got confused. After I had finished the race, I found him ahead of me, wandering around, complaining that he didn't think he was finished when he crossed the finish line, but he didn't know what to do. He'd only finished the first two miles. I could have just sighed and told him that there was nothing he could do. I could have yelled at him for not listening to me when I told him there was a second loop. (But honestly the older I get, the less I yell. It never helps and it only makes people feel bad.) Instead, I took him back on the course and finished the second loop with him.

It was the only way I could think of to fix his mistake. It wasn't terribly fun, because he felt horrible about having an official time that was a "cheat". His legs hurt and so did his tender heart. We walked a few times, but eventually made it back to the finish line. Sam finished the full four miles of the course and we had an approximate time, though we both ducked out of going through the finish a second time since that would only confuse the timers.

The same confusion about the course end happened to Matt the first time he did the Utah Half. I suspect he was dehydrated and that added to the problem, but the race course itself has so many turns and out and backs that it's easy to see how someone could get confused. Matt ended up turning around at an aid station where he should have gone on for another four miles. Instead he got to the finish line, crossed it knowing he hadn't finished thirteen miles, but was not sure what had happened. He was sitting there, waiting for me when I crossed the finish line. When I saw him, I knew something had gone wrong. He told me what had happened, then he sat, despondent for a few minutes, until I told him he had to go back out and finish the race, even if his real race time didn't end up official. At least he would have the satisfaction of knowing he had run all thirteen miles. He completed the race and had satisfaction in knowing he hadn't given up and taken the easy way out. When you can fix it or redo it it's worth the effort.

The next year, Sam did his first triathlon, and again, we made the mistake of not previewing the course, even in a car. It was his first triathlon, and again, we made the mistake of not previewing the course, even in a car. We got in late at night and did not even have time to pick up our packets that evening. We thought we could drive around it the next morning, but we slept in instead and ended up talking to the kids about how to set up a transition area, which was also important. Sam did fine on the run, which is only one loop, but when he hit the bike turn in where he had to decide if he was going back for a second loop or in for the finish, the volunteers guessed—based on the nice bike he was riding (a hand-me-down from me) and the time—that he must be finished and they urged him to the transition area. I found him there after my race, and he was upset and basically paralyzed, feeling there was no point in going to the swim since he hadn't finished the bike.

I tried to talk him into going back on the bike, but he felt like it would be too embarrassing, and everyone else was off the course by then. Besides, he wouldn't get a real time since he'd been sitting there for over ten minutes. Finally, I coaxed him into at least going to the pool and finishing the swim. He'd have the experience of what it was like to move from bike to swim in a reverse triathlon and he could see what his swim time was like and try to beat it the next year. He agreed to this, and he and Matt commiserated with each other again after the race.

The second time Sam did the race, he didn't make that mistake again. I tried to convince Sam that he ought to consider himself lucky. Now that he's made that mistake once, he'll never do it again. If he just keeps going and gets all the mistakes out of the way, then pretty soon he'll be perfect. Sadly, that isn't always true. I've made some mistakes multiple times, like putting my helmet on backwards. I've made at least twice as many mistakes as anyone else in the family, mostly because I've done twice as many races. Just keep in mind that when you're doing a race the first time, your goal needs to be to finish first and foremost. That, in itself, is hard enough amidst all the other newness and confusion.

As a parent, I make a lot of mistakes. My kids make a lot of mistakes, too. But as a kid growing up, I don't remember my parents saying they were sorry to me very many times, and I made a vow as a parent that I wouldn't let my kids grow up thinking their mother was never sorry. I apologize frequently to my kids. More than that, I allow them to criticize my failings and I try to laugh about it. We are all human. I can't always go back and fix everything. I can only apologize and try to do better the next time. I can redo my mistake. In races, as in life, you do the best you can, don't let yourself take the easy way out, and try to do better the next time.

Avoiding Mistakes

Even if you can't avoid all mistakes, it's always nice to avoid as many as you can. Since I've made so many, I can list a lot of the mistakes, and the ways to avoid them for you.

Preview Your Race Course If You Can

After the problems with Sam and Matt getting confused on their course, I realize how important it is to preview a course if you can. I have seen multiple articles on professional races where the lead biker goes off in the wrong direction and leads other bikers astray, only to end up losing the race to a slower biker who didn't go off course because she had either previewed the course in real time or had looked carefully at a map online. For my family, the on-line option has never been as useful as real life. Previewing a course is not just in case you get lost, either. It's also great for training your brain what to expect at each part in the course. I'm not great with directions, and I can get lost even with a GPS in my car. (I have special getting lost super powers.) But previewing race courses regularly has meant that I have never gotten lost in a race.

The first time I tried to preview a race course was when I did my first Ironman. Since I had family in the area I could stay with, I told my coach I could go up weeks before the actual race. He urged me to do so. I drove up from Utah to Coeur D'Alene all by myself at the end of April. It was rainy and cold, nothing like the weather on the day of the race. But it was still a great experience. I brought a map I'd printed out on-line and tried (not very successfully) to keep it dry. I ended up taking a few wrong turns, and using my phone to call for help, but I finally got back to the start and did it all over again to do the full bike course. Then I did a little mini run at the end. The next day, I went down in a wetsuit and got into the freezing cold water just to see what it was like.

When I returned to Utah, I had a huge boost of confidence that I had been able to do the real course. Matt wanted to do his homework before his first Ironman too. He was nervous about the hills on the course in St. George, Utah, which were pretty brutal. So he went down the weekend of his birthday in April as a kind of gift to himself and got a hotel. He did a little bit of the bike the first night, then the rest of it the second day, along with half of the run. He came home warning me about how hard the course was. I probably should have gone with him, but I felt like one of us should stay with the kids, so that was a compromise I made. I had done an Ironman and I figured I would survive.

When we actually drove down to St. George in May, two days before the race to get registered, Matt drove me around the bike and run course and I about died. I understood suddenly what he'd meant about the hills being brutal, and I recalculated my own race goals to account for this. I wasn't going to do anything like what I'd done on my first Ironman course with those kinds of hills on bike and run. In fact, I was almost a full hour slower.

Matt went back in 2012 to do the same thing in preparation for his second Ironman. I elected to stay home again. For Christmas that year I bought myself a CompuTrainer, which is a complex trainer to put your bike on. It calculates your speed and your watts (raw energy output) accurately and works with a heart rate monitor if you want. You can program in your weight and your drag factor to make it feel like you are really outside. To make it even more accurate for training. you can also buy a race course video which will show you the scenery of the course and every turn you will be making on a monitor as you ride. Since I had already done the course in person, it was a useful way to train. In the end, the windy course conditions made the actual day of the race twice as hard as it would have been, but nothing could have prepared me for that. I finished, and thirty percent of the people who started the race didn't. It was the highest DNF (did not finish) rate in the history of Ironman. After that race, they canceled the full Ironman and made it the US Championship race for a half Ironman. Now all the pros can come and try out the super-difficult course.

There are lots of kinds of indoor bikes you can buy now that will allow you to download courses of various races, if you are interested. They can be pricey, I have to warn. The CompuTrainer cost twelve thousand dollars, and that's one thousand dollars more than a standard trainer. However, the watts meter is something that is hard to get and is really very useful. It tells you what energy output you are expending no matter what the course is, so you can compare the output on one course exactly with the output on another. That way you know if your ability to push yourself on the bike is improving even if your times don't show you getting faster per mile because a difficult course required more watts to complete.

Do what you can to preview the course, and then take it easy if you have doubts. Take the corners slowly and look for volunteers to guide you as well as other racers.

Do as Much Race-Specific Training as You Can

It may sound obvious to say that you should try to mimic your race as much as possible in your training, but I am often surprised at how many people ignore this. If your race is going to be uphill a lot, you need to put hills into your training. If it's downhill, you want to mimic that as closely as possible. If it's going to be hot, you should try to make your house as hot as possible. Deena Kastor, who placed third in the Athens Olympics a few years ago, said that the best thing she did in training was to overdress and make herself sweat.[1] She didn't have much time to spend training in the real Athens heat, so she mimicked it as best she could. That's what you want to do as well.

If I know a running race course, I will try to mimic it on my treadmill at home by using zero incline for downhill and punching in up to eight percent for inclines—I've never run a course steeper than that in a race. It's not as good as doing the actual course, but it still helps.

Practice Transitions

If you are doing a triathlon, you need to practice transitions. Practice them a lot. They are the thing that makes triathlon different from anything else. It feels very strange to move from swimming to biking and from biking to running. If you can, find a nearby lake you can swim in. Wear your wetsuit into it, not just your swimming suit. See how it feels to get into the water the first time. Try to force yourself to swim as fast as possible the first hundred yards to give the experience of the race. Then get out of the water, peel out of the wetsuit and RUN toward your bike. See how it feels to try to run when you have just moved from horizontal to vertical. The first race I did this in, I fell down. Twice. I just felt so dizzy.

You need to remember each item that you are going to use for the next discipline and make sure you get it. You also need to remember what items you are going to take off. In my first triathlon, I ended up heading off to get on the bike with my goggles and cap still on. I had to stop, go back to the transition area and take them off, then put on my helmet again, because, well, it didn't fit so good with the goggles on, and the cap would have made me awfully hot if I'd kept it on.

When I am at the end of a swim or a bike, I often remind myself that now is the time to think—not race hard. I ease back a little on my effort level and I start going through a list in my mind of things I need to take off and things I need to put on. This helps me a lot, and these days I almost never forget something I need. In fact, in my last triathlon, one of my goals was to get my transition times down. I was proud of myself because both of my transitions were about thirty seconds, which is a huge im- provement from my first days of racing. Getting transition times down is one of the cheapest ways to get faster in a race. It doesn't cost you a lot of training or heart rate effort. It just requires you to think better, and sometimes to have better gear.

Some gear ideas that will help you go faster in transition include getting a tri suit or something similar. In the first race I did, I found a tight-fitting, mostly Lycra suit that was like a top and shorts only sewn together in the middle so that there was no worry that anything would pull up or float in the water. It worked great. My only complaint about it was that the Lycra wore out too soon and I didn't like to have to climb out of the whole suit with the zipper in the middle if I had to use a porta-potty. So, since then I have moved on to wearing a tri top and tri shorts with a small chamois for biking, but not big enough that it bothers me for the run. Changing outfits in the middle of a race is a pain and it takes a lot of time. The disadvantage of a two piece race outfit is that I have to be careful to put sunscreen on my back in case my top rides up. I've had some bad sunburns on that spot. I wear these same triathlon specific outfits every day I work out. Figure out what you like and wear it for all your training, if possible. Don't waste time changing clothes from discipline to discipline.

Another tip for speed is not wearing socks. Yes, this really works if you have the right bike shoes and running shoes made for triathlon. Triathlon specific shoes have a built-in sock and they go on really fast. If you keep your bike shoes clipped into your bike pedals, you don't have to stop and clip in, either. You just put your bare feet on top of the shoes and start pedaling. Then when you're at speed and can coast for a couple of seconds, tuck your feet in and reach over to pull the strap closed. It takes practice to do this, so don't try to do it for the first time in a race. Once you have mastered this, you're moving forward at twenty miles per hour while your competitor is on his butt in transition putting shoes on. It doesn't save minutes, but it does save seconds. You can put Vaseline along the edge of the run and bike shoes if you find chafing to be a problem. I wear socks in half Ironman-distance races or longer, but not for shorter.

It also helps to have running shoes you don't have to tie. There are various kinds of laces that are elastic and don't need tying, like Lock Laces. Your local running store will have some. They cost a little extra, but I think they're worth it. I don't put on biking gloves while racing, though I wear them in training. I will put on sunglasses if it's hot, but not otherwise. I put on sunscreen before the race starts, so I don't have to stop to do it mid race. If it's a long race, I will sometimes put some small sunscreen packets into my pocket to take out for later use. I put GU packets in my pockets before I get in the water and they usually stay put. Basically, anything you can manage without saves you time.

Train for the End of the Race

I have learned over the years that one of the most important things to train for is the very end of the race. I often find myself running out of energy and trying to figure out how to convince myself to keep pushing. The best thing for this is to do the whole distance in training. This sounds crazy when you are talking about fifty miles or an Ironman, but the closer you can get to it, the better off you are. In 2011, I wanted to really drop time on my fifty mile race, so I did one week of a forty miler on one day followed by a twenty miler the next day.

Let me tell you, I hated that training session more than anything I've ever done. Forty miles on a treadmill, half of it at six percent incline was brutal. I hit a certain point where I could only run at six miles per hour for about three minutes and then I had to walk for three minutes. And getting up the next day to run twenty more miles was really hard on my mind, even more than on my body. I had about six toenails ready to fall off. But I did it. When I hit that point in the race where I want to give up and just walk, I fought back. I knew how to do three minutes on, three minutes off. And it worked. I dropped almost a full hour off my finish time. As they say in the movies—rehearsals are hard, performances are easy. If you do hard training, your races will be easy by comparison. I should add as a proviso here that I did my training runs very slowly, so I didn't hurt myself in training. I made the distance the goal, not the time. Just covering the distance in as close to the real terrain as possible is the best thing to aim for.

Preparing for Weather

It helps to be ready for any weather during a race. I have a couple of races that are in spring or fall and for those you never know what to expect. I bring a set of warm clothes that I put on first and then gradually add layers until I feel comfortable. Then just before the race starts, I peel down one layer because I always warm up while racing. And no matter what the weatherman says, I prepare for snow, hail, sleet, and rain.

One year, I signed up to do my annual fifty-miler, and every weekend before the race it was raining or snowing. I just did not want to go outside in that weather for hours on end to train, so I stayed indoors. Yes, I ended up not knowing the course as well as I wished I had, but I don't regret training indoors. There is only so much unpleasantness I can take. I can deal with hail during a race but I don't want it every day. I did go out once with a supposedly waterproof jacket and after an hour I had cold water dripping down my back, and I was shivering badly. So I didn't do that again. There are times when it is just not worth it. Prepare the best you can, and let that be enough.

The Day Before

I would not recommend doing a lot of training on the course the day before a race. I think you should probably be sitting at home or by the pool side, resting. I see people out doing hills on Ironman the day before, and I guess they are just tougher than I am. There's a time and a place for race specific training, and it's not the day before. If you aren't ready for the hills or the distance, the day before a race is not the day to prepare.

Setting Up Your Transition

If you take the time to set up your transition carefully, you will save time and frustration.

Most triathletes bring a towel to transition, not so much to actually dry off on, but to simply mark a space in transition that is their own, and to help guide them to that place. A brightly colored towel is a good idea, and I recommend running through transition once or twice before the race begins to make sure you can spot your towel.

If your bike is assigned a rack position, find it and work from there. If you are in a race that does not have assigned rack positions, think about where you want to be. Do you prefer having your bike close to the entry or to the exit? If you place it near the exit, you will be with most of the fastest triathletes, which may or may not be what you want. You will probably face more competition for spots there and will have to go early to get them. You may also face people trying to get a spot and pushing your stuff around. Please be calm about this. There is usually space for another bike.

Once you have your bike on the rack (hanging by the saddle either way works, though some races want you to alternate to fit more bikes in), spread out your towel. You will be wearing your swim suit or tri suit, if you've got one, to the race. So hang up your wetsuit on the rack temporarily while you set up your other gear. You will want to put your bike shoes out, if you have some. If not, put out your running shoes with socks tucked into the shoes loosely.

Also set up your helmet in a way that is easy to put on, usually face down. Practice grabbing it a few times and putting it on. If you have sunglasses or gloves, put them inside the helmet so they are easy to find. If you need fuel for a longer race, put your GU packets out so you can grab them easily. Hopefully you are wearing a tri suit with some pockets for this sort of thing. I will often put GU packets into my tri suit before I get into the water, so I have less to think about, but it can be a little less comfortable in the swim.

Set up your running shoes and socks separately from your biking shoes and socks, if you have separate shoes. Normally, once you have your socks on, you will leave that pair on. More advanced triathletes race without socks entirely so they don't have to take the extra time to pull socks on wet feet. But beginners probably will want to have the comfort of their usual socks. It depends on if it is worth saving thirty seconds to you to skip that part of transition.

Sometimes I will have a small cooler chest on my towel with my fuel belt in it, frozen so that I can drink cold fluid during the run in a long half Ironman that doesn't have good aid stations. A full length Ironman will provide plenty of fuel and you won't need to worry about it unless you are very particular about what you take in. I also keep little packets of sunscreen to tuck into my tri suit so that if I start to feel a burn on the run, I can reapply the sunscreen easily. On a long race, I may also bring ChapStick.

Step back from your towel once you have set things up and see if it makes sense to you. When you come in from the swim, you will take the wetsuit off while standing on your towel. Hang it on the bike rack to drip dry or if you have a bucket for your wetsuit, you can put it in there. You will see people with buckets. That's what they're for. Don't waste too much time drying off. Put on your helmet and shoes and go.

The last hundred yards of a swim, I start thinking about what I need to do in T1 (transition from swim to bike). I think: wetsuit off, helmet on, shoes on. Or whatever variation I'm going to do. Wetsuit off, helmet and sunglasses on, shoes and socks on. I just say it over and over again until I've got everything on and am ready to move to the bike exit. There will be a zone designated for you to mount the bike. Don't mount until then. Don't worry if it takes you a few seconds to get on. Just let people get by you if they're faster.

The last part of the bike, I do the same thing, reminding myself what I need to do to get through T2 (transition from bike to run). I think: helmet off, bike shoes off, running shoes on. Or: helmet off, sunglasses off, race belt with number on, running shoes on. Sometimes I don't bike with the race number on because it flaps in the wind and my bike is already marked, but I have to put it on before I run, or I face disqualification. When you're out on the run, you don't have to think about any more transitions, just the finish line. If you do some walking, make sure you cross the finish line running so you can have a nice photo. Then you get to go back to the transition zones and pick everything up.

You will have to get everything you brought to the race back into your car. Get some bags big enough to fit everything into and still carry easily. I have a giant tri backpack that will even fit my helmet. Some races make you bike from a parking spot to the transition area for a couple miles. Think of it as a warm-up. Some races will offer you the option of putting shoes at the water's edge. If this happens, bring a pair of shoes you don't care about and can get into when dripping wet. If you are new to triathlon, you will want those shoes because the offer means the run to the transition area is painful, rocky, and dangerous.

How to Put a Wetsuit On

Once you are set up it's time to get into that wetsuit.

If you have purchased a wetsuit online, you will get it in the mail and stare at it, wondering what in the world you are supposed to do to get *that* on your body. Hopefully, you have some anti-chafing lubricant like BodyGlide on hand. If not, go buy some before you try it on. And yes, do try it on before race day, to make sure you can get into it. Apply BodyGlide to your ankles, all the way to about halfway up your shins. Also apply it to your arms around your wrists and around the back of your neck where the wetsuit fastens to avoid nasty chafing there.

If you are wearing a watch during the race, take it off to apply BodyGlide and to get your wetsuit on. Then put it on and tuck it under your wetsuit so it stays on after you have taken the wetsuit off. If you have to put on a timing chip, also put that on after you have your wetsuit on. I have seen people at races wearing them outside the wetsuit and underneath. I wear mine underneath so I don't have to worry about putting it back on in transition. One more thing in transition can be one too many. I have lots of stories about things that I have forgotten in transition and have just had to live without or had to go back for and waste all that time.

Now that you have your BodyGlide on, it's time to get into that wetsuit.

Put the legs of the wetsuit on first. You are going to poke your foot through by gently pushing it as far as you can into the wetsuit leg and then wiggling and tugging and inching up the material until it is around your ankle. Then you do the same with the other leg, so that both ankles are in. Then bend over and pull up the wetsuit in folds until it is up around your knees on both sides. Work it up from there to your thighs. For me, my wetsuit reaches all the way to my ankles. For some people, it will end up a little above your ankle, depending on how tall you are and what size suit you have.

Once you have the wetsuit up around your butt and it fits your crotch, you can work on putting your arms in. Arms are easier than legs, but it's a similar process, tugging and then pulling it up so that there aren't any wrinkles.

It will feel tight. You will feel pressure. This is normal. It may feel like it is hard to breathe, but if you can get the wetsuit on, you are doing fine. The hardest part is now to get it zipped closed. After many years, I have figured out how to do this on my own, most of the time. But don't be surprised if some random stranger asks you to help do the final zip up the back. And don't feel uncomfortable asking for help from another triathlete. You can make a friend and chat about the race or just ask for help. No obligation. Or if you have a support person, ask them to help do the final zip up the back. There will be a string dangling. Don't worry about it. Now you're in. Good job.

Endnotes

1. Joe I. Vigil, "The Anatomy of a Medal," *Cool Running*, 2013, http://www.coolrunning.com/engine/2/2_1/the-anatomy-of-a-medal.shtml.

CHAPTER 8

THE WORST SUMMER EVER

During the winter following my first Ironman, I listened to my children complain about everything athletic they were required to do in school, in particular the dreaded one mile run. It wasn't that I didn't get it. I did. I remember nothing so clearly as hating running the mile run in my own school days. I hated PE in junior high school. One of the reasons I joined the swim team in high school was to get out of regular PE and avoid the one mile run. Not only was it difficult for me to run a mile because I was a little chubby in elementary school and junior high school, but it was also humiliating to do it badly.

For years I thought my lack of success in sports was because I wasn't born athletic. But after I had done my first Ironman, I looked back and realized that the real reason I struggled so badly was only that I hadn't been properly trained. I didn't run on a regular basis. I didn't know how it felt to run easily, or how to breathe while running. I didn't know how to reduce the pain in my shoulders which came because I tightened my fists and gritted my teeth. I didn't know how to pace myself. I didn't know how to eat properly before a run. I didn't have the proper shoes for running, and on, and on.

I decided my kids were going to benefit from a mother who now knew a lot more about proper athletic training. If you want elementary and junior high school kids to be able to run a mile without stopping, you have to get them to run more than once a year in the actual race. This seems obvious, doesn't it? I suppose that somehow PE teachers are hoping that these kids run in other activities in their lives, but it isn't true anymore, if it ever was. It certainly isn't true for any of my kids.

I do have the younger ones walk to and from the elementary school (one mile round trip) and they complain about it bitterly. Most of the parents in our neighborhood drive their kids to school and pick them up every day. They feel that this is a safety issue, so that their children are not kidnapped. I don't want my kids taken any more than anyone else. But what is a greater risk to children in our current day and age? Being kidnapped or becoming obese because of a sedentary lifestyle? It seems obvious to me that it is the latter. So, I teach my kids safety rules, and they walk.

Bribery Is a Great Tool

If your kids are into soccer or football or basketball, they probably do plenty of running. If they're into piano, violin, or the chess club, probably not. You are going to have to intervene, and you're going to have to do it cleverly. Even my two most social kids, Sage and Zach, don't like team sports. The other three are all geeky home bodies interested mostly in academics. If your kids are like mine and fun isn't a reason to do sports, think of other reasons they may buy into. For my kids, they were interested in training in part because I was already doing it and in part because the way I talked about triathlon was more cerebral. Still, I knew I was going to have to bring in the big guns: bribes.

Hope (thirteen at this point) said she would rather swim a mile every day than run it. I told her that didn't count, since she was still going to have to run a mile in PE at the junior high since they didn't have a pool, and it was a test that had been standardized so they knew exactly what her fitness level was for a mile run, not the mile swim. Sam (ten) and Sage (eleven) were more naturally athletic. But Faith (seven) and Zach (five) were concerns of mine. Faith was capable of running and understanding what I explained about the principles, but she was also youngest sister of three. She thought then, and continues to think now, that if she cannot do anything as well as Sage and Hope are doing it, she has failed. I had to keep this in mind when planning runs. I had to make sure that Faith focused on her own improvements, not on comparisons. Zach was still a baby in my mind. While he loved running, he tended to have a very short attention span. For this reason, the track was an excellent place for him. He could sit in the grassy middle of the track and watch us. I could watch him and make sure he was safe. And when he wanted to, he could join in.

Every summer since my kids were small, I have worked hard to make the summer a great learning experience. I've read books about how kids lose so much during the summer when they're not in school. Well, not in my house. Even when I struggled with money, we would go to the library to check out math and science books the kids could read and work through. One year, Matt offered the kids a prize to go through all the *StarCraft* missions so they could play with him. If they finished all the missions, they got to go out to dinner with Dad at a special place at the end of the summer. Anyone who finished could go, and Matt made sure to make that dinner sound like a really great prize. At the time, we rarely went out to eat, so it was a big deal to the kids. Sage eventually asked if she could do something else because computer games didn't interest her, so Matt let her choose reading a complete Encyclopedia instead. They all went out to Denny's for dinner; the kids thought that was the best thing ever.

I usually let the kids choose a goal for the summer and then help them work toward it. As a reward for these goals, when the kids were younger, we would go out shopping for treats each week. One year Sam got these horrible giant gummy sharks that he thought were great. I tasted one and thought they were terrible, but it was his choice, not mine. It motivated him.

In later years, there have been larger goals and much larger rewards to be worked towards. Sometimes the project itself is the reward, like the year I helped the kids write, direct, and perform a neighborhood play with a couple dozen friends. I try to make sure that the kids have some say in their summer project, but there are times when I nudge them in a particular direction and then try to make sure the reward makes it worth their while. I also try to back off if it really seems like it's going badly. That said, "the worst summer ever" is the one when I tried to turn all of my kids into runners. I can't say they liked it, but they all gave it a try and I think it forced them to see that running, even if it isn't their favorite thing, was not as bad as they had first believed.

Teach Your Kids HOW to Run

The summer of 2007, I announced that our family summer project was going to be running every day. Yes, every day, at least a mile, so that they got over their fear of running the mile. Now, telling kids who cannot fathom running a mile that they have to run a mile every day or even three times a week is likely to create a rebellion. It did at our house. It's no wonder school gym coaches don't like to go through that on a regular basis. But if they did it more often, it might actually decrease the bad reaction. I also think running with kids can help motivate them, though perhaps it's unreasonble to expect PE teachers to do that all day long.

To get kids to hurt less when they run, you actually have to get them to run more, but in smaller doses. My recommendation—quarter mile sprints to start with. Then increase to longer distances like a half mile or mile, teaching them how to relax while running so they don't cramp up. Show them how to keep their pace easy enough at the beginning so that they can push hard at the finish line. They should be able to hold a conversation during most easy running. They need to find a pace that they can feel comfortable at, like they can go forever. And you as the parent should be aware that at first, or even possibly for a long time, that pace might mean alternating one minute of running and one minute of walking or four minutes of running and two minutes of jogging. No matter what anyone tells your children, you need to reassure them that they don't have to run every second of that mile run, even in a race. Watch any real marathon or Ironman race and you will see that some of the best runners will walk through aid stations. And the people who are more middle of the road runners do a lot more walking because it helps them keep going farther, and that's the point.

As their endurance increases, hopefully you can get your kids to run more than one mile, even two or three miles at a stretch, very slowly. This will help build their aerobic system. Long runs are one of the corner stones of all distance training. There is also a significant psychological effect, because, if you know how it feels to run several miles, one mile doesn't seem so hard to wrap your mind around anymore. When you hear a child say for the first time, "It's only a mile," that is music to your ears. Now that my kids have been training for a half marathon (more than thirteen miles) that one mile run in the gym seems easy. But I'm getting ahead of myself.

Many kids feel pressed in PE classes to go harder, faster, but as far as I can tell, the only result of this is kids pushing themselves to their utter limit in the first quarter mile and then feeling like they are going to die. Defeated, they walk the rest of the run and feel terrible. If they simply ran at an easy pace at the beginning, then got faster as they got closer to the finish line, they would finish with a sense of accomplishment and even a runner's high.

In my experience, children want to do well. Teach children to listen to their own bodies as much as possible as a gauge for their own abilities.

It is unreasonable to expect someone who is untrained and out of shape to be able to run for a full mile in the first place. Not even at a very slow pace. When I do training plans for people, one of the first things I ask is how fast they can run a mile because it's a great measure of their fitness. If they can't run it, they can still get on a treadmill or go outside and figure out how long it takes to walk a mile. It's not meant to be humiliating. It's just a starting point, so that you know what a reasonable improvement over a few months of training will be. If you can only walk the mile at three miles per hour, that's OK. That's your starting point. You'll move up from there. Some people need to lose weight before they can reasonably run, so they'll do walking for up to a year before they add in running. They need to know that's OK. As the parent/coach, you need to give positive feedback to whatever attempts are made.

With kids, you can expect some resistance. Let me describe what happened at my house when I suggested my summer running plan. There was a massive outcry. They moaned and groaned. They told me I was the worst mom ever. They still think this summer of running was horrible and when I told my kids that I was planning to write about it in this book, Sam said, "Tell everyone never to do that. It was the worst summer ever." So there aren't fond memories on their side. I got over it. I told them what I expected. I told them I would give rewards, as always. And then every morning I announced it was time to go running and that they would need to get shoes and running clothes on.

The truth is, of course, I couldn't make them run with me. Some of the older ones, I couldn't even have forced to get in the car with me. But I put them into a situation in which they might as well just do it and get it over with. I told them sternly I expected them to come, and Matt backed me up. Then I offered them bribes, small treats every day and larger ones at the end of the summer. That was enough to get them to try running, to see if they liked it. I had fairly low standards. I just wanted them not to hate it and to maybe have a few experiences where it felt good to move their bodies as runners. I was there to listen to their breathing, and to tell them if they were going too hard. Mostly that was my job, to tell them to slow down and enjoy it a little more. That's good advice for everyone.

Keep Records

I have been keeping a training log for nearly eight years now. It's not expensive. It's not complicated. I wait until I can get lined, spiral bound notebooks at Walmart for ten cents each. I use them for brainstorming writing projects and for my training logs. I keep my log on my writing desk next to my computer at my left side. I write simply the date to the upper left, and then what I did and the time. For example Jan. 11, 2002 — bike 1:00. That's pretty basic, but if I feel like it I add in more information. It can be either objective or subjective. If I know exactly how many miles I went, I can put that in, or I can note my heart rate. I can also put in if I felt sick that day, or if it felt hard, or if I felt great. Sometimes I write in only that I was too sick to work out, nothing more than that.

Over the last eight years, I have filled about four notebooks, one week on each page. I keep special track of my races, which I circle and can look back at when I do the same race the next year. I like to see tiny little improvements — and when I say tiny, I mean tiny. Even one second off means it is a PR (personal record) and that is something to celebrate, especially as I get older.

I also like to measure myself against a fairly simple one-hour running test. I do this one of two ways. The first way is to try to run as far as possible. The second is to try to keep my heart rate on average below 140 and see how far I can go. One heart beat lower on average or a tenth of a mile faster are both significant improvements. Maybe I am a geek to care about these things, but I think that my attention to detail helps keep me motivated. Even if I use a treadmill at the gym, I can see if I'm improving by looking at the estimate of calories burned. If I can burn one more calorie in a fifteen minute mini-workout, I know that I've worked harder than I worked the last time I was on the machine. I have the evidentiary proof.

I don't only keep track of my cardio workouts. I also write in weight lifting workouts twice a week. I keep track of reps and weights for each muscle I'm working. I also keep track of yoga time spent. I think yoga is a great way to become attuned to your body and also to deal with trouble areas and avoid injuries.

At the end of the week, I will add up my hours in each discipline (bike, run, swim, and yoga/weights) and then I have a quick way to see how hard the week was for me. A week that I've done more than ten hours of training in is moderate, more than fifteen is really difficult, less than ten is usually an easy week or a race week.

It doesn't matter where you start. If you can only do ten minutes a day, just keep track of it so that you can see the minutes piling up. If you'd rather use an electronic device to help keep track, you can go online and find apps that are available for free. MyFitnessPal app is free and available on the iPhone. You can log your calorie intake as well as calories burned and reference this whenever you want. My husband uses a GPS watch and downloads the data from the recorder onto his computer. I still think my notebook is cheaper and easier, but to each his own.

With my kids, I decided I wanted them to see their progress visually. So the first day we went, I brought a notebook to record times for each child. I wanted to know a baseline for them to start on, and then they could move up from there. Writing things down isn't to make anyone feel bad. No one else ever needs to see it. For my kids, I tried to make sure they understood I only wanted them to be able to be proud of themselves. I also explained to them that not every day is a good day. Some days you are sick. Some days you are stressed. Some days you feel yucky for completely inexplicable reasons. That's OK. You have permission to have a bad day now and again. Just keep going and you'll improve.

We did quarter mile runs (one full lap of the track) because I thought that was short enough they could really sprint. I used my watch as a stop watch. I ran at a slow pace for me (about ten to eleven minutes per mile) alongside them and tried to encourage the kids verbally. I didn't stand on the sideline and just time my kids and tell them to keep going. When you have five kids, they are all going to be at different paces, so you can't expect them all to run together. I would run with one kid for one lap, then hang back and run with another kid the next lap and so on. Every once in a while, if we did a 100 yard dash, I would really go at full speed to give them someone to compete against.

That summer Sage seemed particularly gifted at running. She had a naturally good running stride, and a slim build. She could run faster than anyone else (although Faith tried to keep up with her for the first hundred meters of every lap). She also tended to look the worst after she pushed herself hard, a pale face, sweat dripping down her forehead. She loved it. Go figure.

I still have the notebook I kept for that year. I started out using a heart rate monitor on one kid at a time, because I had found a heart rate monitor useful for me in training, not to make me work harder, but to teach me what it felt like when I went at the proper paces for different distances and to make sure that I didn't ever go too hard on longer races. What I found was that a heart rate monitor was essentially useless for children. Instead we used a scale to gauge effort level from 1 to 10. A 100 yard sprint was a 10. A quarter mile sprint was an 8. A two mile run/walk was about a 4. This helped the kids get the feel of different training speeds.

I also mixed up the workouts. On Mondays, we always did sprints of a quarter mile or less. On Wednesdays, we did a one mile run test experience. On Fridays, we did long runs of two to three miles. The kids hated Fridays at the beginning, but came to like them more and more because I did not try to get them to run at any particular pace. I let them walk as much as they wanted to. It was just a matter of how long it would take if they ran the whole thing to get home. They usually ran some of it, but if they didn't, we just waited until they were finished. I counted laps with them, and encouraged them. I also noticed that Hope, Sam, and Faith tended to walk together. That was great for their relationships as siblings.

Lest you think it was all roses, however, one day it rained terribly and Faith was just so upset by the rain and so grouchy that she sat down in the middle of the track and refused to move out of anyone's way. She shivered there and wouldn't go out to the car on my suggestion or even put on her coat. She wanted to make good and sure that I knew how unpleasant the day was for her. She cried pitifully and I wondered if anyone else was going to come to the track and see what was going on and call DCFS for torturing my seven-year-old. Eventually, the rest of us finished and we got in the car.

I seriously wondered if I had done the right thing. I began to second guess my strict plan of running three days a week. After that day, I tried some other activities, like running in the neighborhood or biking on a local trail as a family instead. I think these days were just as useful. There are times when it's great to take off your watch and just run for the fun of running, just to feel what running is like, to rejoice in the way your body moves. I believe in record keeping, but I try not to take it too far.

Rewards for Outcome and Effort

For the running summer, I set up two alternate reward systems— one based on outcome and one based purely on effort. I think the best motivations for kids include some of each of these. You want to encourage kids who are not naturally talented to keep trying—

because who knows, you may be surprised down the road. But you also want to encourage the kids who show real, concrete results that are measurable, so that it's not just a game to make it "seem" like they are working hard.

For our summer of running, I decided that any kid who could run the mile in under ten minutes on the track would get a reward at the end of the summer of twenty dollars. For under nine minutes, the reward would be fifty dollars, for under eight minutes, one hundred dollars. Some of my kids are really motivated by monetary rewards. Sage is one of them, so this really interested her.

For the other kids, I brought more immediate rewards, both during our training and afterward. If you are working really hard, you have to be careful what kind of foods you try to eat. If it's too heavy, you may end up throwing it back up. So light carbs, things like crackers or fruits are good. My kids were intrigued by Gatorade and GU, which are things that I eat mostly when I am training really long and hard for an Ironman or other ultra distance event. But perhaps because these were forbidden treats, the kids seemed motivated to earn them by running. I brought a few GU packets for them to try while running and plenty of Gatorade in bottles.

I don't see anything dangerous in GU, it's just sugar, but it costs a dollar a pouch and it's not real food, so that was the only time they got it. Some kids liked it more than others. The ones who didn't like it had crackers, and there was water if they didn't like the aftertaste or salt in Gatorade. There were always water bottles and snacks at the end of each quarter mile to be picked up and consumed as you walked a little in the next quarter mile. Now and again, when we did a long run, I promised to take everyone out for an ice cream cone at a local fast food restaurant on the way home.

One of the most memorable days that summer was a Saturday when Matt decided to come to the track with us and see what the story was. He had heard complaints from kids and glowing reports from me because I could see the improvements in them very quickly. I should say that at this point, Matt hadn't done much training himself. He did a little running now and then, maybe a 5k or two, but he wasn't into triathlon. The kids generally associated athletics with me and not with him. That Saturday on the track, we had a one mile race. The seven of us all lined up together, and Matt and I set our watches. The kids soon got to see that even though I could beat Dad in a race of any distance longer than a 5k, there was no way I could compare to his speed on a single lap of the track. He was at least twenty seconds ahead of me. The only person who could keep up with Matt appeared to be Sage. She was breathing hard and struggling desperately, but she pushed harder and harder. I realized when I checked my watch, that in the first half mile, she was ready to go under seven minutes for her mile. She slowed down a little for the second lap, and then, suddenly, about ten yards from the finish line, she collapsed.

I hurried over to her and tried to convince her that she had the energy to keep walking the last ten yards. She was so close to going under eight minutes and getting that hundred-dollar prize, but she refused for at least a minute to get up. At last, she ended up finishing in about 9:30, ahead of all the other kids, but not as well as she could have done. I talked for some time afterward in the car and at home about pacing yourself properly and leaving a little for the last part of the race. I think I ended up giving her the fifty-dollar prize anyway, since she had been so close. Sam, Hope, and Faith got twenty dollars each. Zach didn't care about money, and was perfectly happy with a piece of candy for the random running around the track.

Keep It Fun, and Do It Together

If you want your kids to do something, do it with them. When Hope was struggling with playing the violin at age eight, I ended up getting myself an inexpensive full size violin, and I learned how to play violin with her. It taught me a lot about music for one thing, but it was also a chance for the kids to see that I struggled too. I wasn't just Mom; I was a person just like they were. And it gave us time to spend together doing something we had in common. All great reasons for parents and kids to do something—whatever it is they choose—together.

These days, people will ask me how I get grouchy teenagers to go out running in the middle of winter. Well, the simple answer is: I run with them. I talk and chat and make it fun. I encourage them when they feel like they can't keep going. I make achievable goals, and I never ever yell at them. I can hear their breathing next to me. I can tell when they are about to collapse, and I will walk with them so they don't. It has not been my experience that teens don't want to spend time with their parents. Yes, they want parents to disappear when their friends are around. But my teens—and I think most kids—desperately want the attention and approval of their parents. They don't want their parents to tell them what to do, but if you are willing to do what they want to do, or to help them achieve a goal that they have, then they will gladly stay with you.

This is one of the most important lessons for inspiring your children to do something. You do it with them. If you want your children to learn how to cook, don't buy them a cookbook. Bring them into the kitchen with you, explain every step and give them something to do. Even at a young age, this is a great principle. I remember when Hope was about eighteen months old, Matt used to sit her up on the counter in our kitchen and crack eggs. She was thrilled to watch him do it, and slowly, he let her take charge of the problem herself. He let her tap the egg on the counter, then he opened it. And finally, he let her crack the eggs herself. Before she was two, she was great at cracking eggs, because it was a fun thing to do with Dad.

Because Sage had shown the least hatred of running, I asked her in the summer of 2007 if she might be interested in running a 5k with me. She had been the only one of the three kids to complete a three mile run on the track in less than thirty minutes, which to me is a kind of threshold of running vs. jogging. I told her that there was a 5k on the weekend of July 4 in a nearby town, and that I would run the race with her. I had done the same race the year before on my own, and it was well run and inexpensive, plus the money went to a literacy cause that I believed in. Sage agreed to come and do it with me, so this was going to be my first ever experience actually racing *with* one of my kids.

We drove to the race just the two of us, chatted about school and friends, and then got to the starting line. It took a few seconds before the mass of people let us start moving, then, slowly we were able to run. The first part of the course was downhill, and I figured that my main job was to keep Sage from going too fast and giving up halfway through the race.

The first third of the course was easy, downhill, through the center of town, past the high school, and then the tiny movie theater. Sage and I felt like we were in a big crowd of people who all had the same purpose we did. It was a beautiful summer day, and, since it was about 8:00 a.m., it wasn't too hot yet. There is something amazing about the beginning of a race with so many people on a holiday like the Fourth of July, a special energy that comes from knowing the rest of the day is going to be spent with family and friends, and that you will be up late that night watching fireworks and making memories.

The second third of the course was straight uphill into the Wasatch Mountains to the east, and that was where Sage began to struggle. She looked sick and pale and started to shake and sweat. I was starting to get nervous that she was going to collapse again like she had on the track. I told her it was time to walk, so she walked the rest of the way up the hill. When we turned and were on flat again, we started a slow jog to the finish line. We stopped one more time. Once I pointed out the finish line, Sage sped ahead of me, and I let her cross just before me. She was pretty tired immediately afterward, and just laid down on the ground for about twenty minutes. But then, when we got back in the car together, she was very chatty. She was proud of herself and wore the race t-shirt on Saturdays for months afterward to show it off. She was the only one of the kids who had done a full 5k, which was a nice bragging right.

At the end of the summer in 2007, it was time for the other kids to have their chance at the Striders Memorial Day Run. Matt signed up to run the 5k with some buddies at his office. I was running the half marathon. After Sage's success at the Fourth of July 5k, the other kids decided they wanted to try a race, albeit a shorter one. So the next year, in May of 2008, we signed the kids up for the Striders Memorial Day Run. Matt signed up to run the 5k with some buddies at his office. I was running the half marathon. All the kids came, and Hope watched them while Matt and I raced. Then it was time for the one-mile kid race. Even Zachary was signed up to run.

Matt took on the older kids, and I was in charge of getting Zach and Faith to the finish line. The venue was beautiful, out by the Great Salt Lake on a trail that runs through the length of Davis County. The park there has a pond full of ducks and swans, along with seagulls overhead. The kids' race was just around the pond and past it toward the cornfields, and it was lovely. But it was a lot different with the younger kids than it had been with Sage.

At first, I had a hard time because Zach kept sprinting ahead of us and then I had to talk Faith into catching up to him. She resented being beaten and she didn't like running much, either. I coaxed and prodded, trying to tell her she didn't want her little brother beating her while trying to keep Zach in sight. It's easier when you only have one kid to help with a race, but that's not the way it always is in real life. Sometimes you have to deal with different needs, and you do the best you can.

The course was an out and back, and when we hit the turn-around, Zach started to be the one who didn't want to continue. He just wanted to sit by the sidewalk and do it later. I didn't think that was a good plan because I thought he might be trampled. I also wanted to be with him when he finished, so he could feel triumphant. I kept him going by holding his hand. I reminded him of the cool medal he would get at the finish line and of the treats that he could have from the food table. "There are donuts," I said, "and all you have to do is keep going."

Finally, at the finish line, there was a moment when both Faith and Zach got excited to see their time overhead on the timer, and they could see kids getting medals just past the finish. They sprinted ahead, and I told myself that the race was a great cool down for my half marathon.

Training with Different Ability Levels

In 2012, with much older kids, we had some bigger plans. Matt talked the kids into signing up for his company's annual half marathon, the Salt Lake Half, in April. I wrote up training plans for all of them (except for Zach, who showed no interest and is probably still too young for thirteen miles). The result?

Most of them followed the training plans for a few weeks, and then lost interest. Sam was more diligent because he was working toward a Scout Fitness Badge and he had to check off every day of training in order to earn it. It's really hard for kids—even teens—to think of doing a two to three hour workout every week that hurts and pushes them past their comfort levels. And then there was the problem that everyone was training at different paces and with different styles.

Sam could run straight through without needing walking breaks at about five miles per hour or faster. Some Saturdays it worked out that he could run with Matt, who was training for an Ironman at a fairly slow pace. But other times he tried to talk Hope into going out with him. But Hope could only run at a five mile per hour pace for four minutes and then she had to walk for two minutes. That annoyed Sam. Sage was doing the same run four minutes, walk two minutes plan, but she ran at a faster pace than Hope did and walked faster, too. I know, because I went out for about ten miles trying to get the two of them to stay together. It was hard. Sage felt like going so slowly made her feet hurt more. And Hope ended up falling back if I tried to keep up with Sage's natural pace. Faith, on the other hand, wasn't running at all. She just hated it and even if we ran for only three minutes, she would sound out of breath and like she was about to die. She struggles with asthma, and I didn't want to press her too hard.

So, eventually, we realized that all the kids were going to have to go at their own paces. I ended up training with all of them at various times. Sometimes Hope would do her long workout on Wednesdays with me. Then she would walk ten miles or so with Faith on the weekends. One Saturday I ended up running my own workout in preparation for the half marathon, twelve miles at a 7:45 pace on the treadmill. Then I ran Sage's ten miles with her about six hours later. And right after that, I walked nine miles with Faith. That was six hours of working out for me, and my legs really hurt afterward. But, it was more important that my kids felt like I wanted to be with them and was willing to sacrifice what my training needs were to make sure that they had someone to chat with while training.

Tips to Make Workouts Fun for Kids

Workout with Them at Their Pace

Don't try to push them to go as fast as you want to go. Of course, once they are faster than you, then you will have to find someone else to run at their pace.

Talk While You're Running

Talk about the running or talk about anything. Ask your kids questions. Wait for them to answer. Sometimes you will wait a while. That's OK. They want to see if you really care what they have to say. Take them seriously. Listen. Take their side of things. Believe them when they tell you what their life is like. Tell them about when you were a teenager. Have a sense of humor about how different life is now.

Have a Plan and a Back-up Plan

If you are out with your kids, know how far you intend to go. Make sure that your child has trained well enough to be able to go this far or plan that they will go a distance that is right for them. Make it clear if you expect them to wait for you to finish. Have them bring a book or something else to do. Or make arrangements for a pickup from someone else. And if your child looks like he/she is struggling, make a quick change to the plan while assuring him/her it's not because you have given up on the plan completely, it just needs to be adjusted. Walking is fine if you need to get the distance completed.

Offer a Reward

This can be a reward immediately after the workout for younger children or a more distant reward later, like dinner out with Dad and Mom the day before the race. Also be sure that you only offer the reward to the children who are doing the workout. Yes, this can cause some weeping and wailing, but it isn't fair to the child who is doing the workout to not get a special reward.

Put on a Good Face

Even if you are struggling, try to pretend you aren't for the sake of your children. Make them believe you are having fun. Joke around. It might even turn out to make you feel better, too. You can tell your kids how unpleasant you find it another time, if you feel the need to be honest.

Buy Them the Proper Gear When They are Ready for It

You can make this a reward to look forward to, or as a kind of rite of passage. I don't spend a lot of money on kids doing short runs, but when they've proven to me they are serious by following a training plan for about a month, I will shell out real money for expensive shoes and racing gear.

Sign Them Up for Races

Get signed up to race, then make the races fun. Go out to dinner beforehand. Think about going to a hotel that's close to the race venue to make a mini-vacation out of it. Buy some souvenirs from the race so they remember it fondly.

Make a Competition

You will have to be sensitive about which kids will like this and which won't. Not all kids want a competition, but you can make it a friendly one by giving rewards equally to all who participate. You can also offer handicaps. One thing Matt sometimes does is try to beat the kids by half. He will do fifteen miles and they do ten miles and try to beat him. Then they feel like it's doable and focus on it. He never lets them win on purpose. It's always a real competition. The kids know if they beat their Dad, they did it fair and square They also know that next time, he will change the rules, if he needs to, so he has a chance.

Hand Out Compliments

Tell them everything they did well, even the tiniest of things. In general, I don't think parents give enough positive feedback to their kids. This can make kids have the feeling that nothing they do is right. Be especially careful of this while training with kids. Don't give them too much advice at once. Wait for them to ask for it. And load them up with good feelings about what they have done. It will make them want to come back for more. Don't be insincere. Make sure your compliments are real. Your children will know.

Dream Big

Matt has started to talk to Sam about doing an Ironman together as soon as Sam turns eighteen. It seems really crazy right now to think about it since he is only fifteen, but talking about it and making plans for what bike Sam will ride makes everything about racing seem like more fun.

CHAPTER 9

HOW TRIATHLON SAVED MY MARRIAGE

M ost people have seen the inspiring video of Julie Moss at the 1982 Ironman Hawaii Championships where she falls down the last one hundred meters of the run and is passed, then crawls to the finish line to take second. If there is anything that shows more about the human spirit and the lengths it will go to conquer the weakness of the body, I have yet to see it. I watched the video a couple of times when I was in high school, but it didn't make me say—Hey, I want to do that race. It made me say—Julie Moss is crazy and so are all the people who do Ironman. I was intent on staying away from a sport that looked like it might well kill you.

Even when I did my first couple of Olympic distance races in 2004, I wasn't thinking Ironman. Ironman was for real athletes, not people like me. Ironman was for, well, Ironmen. Right? But after I'd done one, that all changed. And it didn't just change for me. Some people still think I'm crazy, and that just because I can do an Ironman doesn't mean anyone else can. But the people who

know me well, know that I'm simply determined, not particularly stronger or more naturally gifted than anyone else. And I've
started to think of myself as being a lot like Julie Moss. If I were
doing an Ironman and I fell down that close to the finish line, you
bet that I would crawl to the end. I would not let someone take me
off the course to get medical attention, not when I was that close.
Finishing Ironman is something special, and the closer you are
to someone who has done one, the more the inspiration rubs off.

If You Can Do It, So Can I

I did my first Utah Half Ironman (1.2 mile swim, 56 mile bike,
13.1 mile run) in August 2007. Matt came and watched the entire
race. He left the kids with my sister who lives in Provo. This was
the first time he had really been able to watch an entire race from
beginning to end from the sidelines, not just from video footage.
He'd come to see me finish races, and had even cheered me on at
the Ironman, but he'd never seen the whole guts of it. He brought
a book to read, but I don't think he ended up spending any time
reading. There were always people to watch, to cheer on, and
things to learn from what they were doing, both right and wrong.

When Matt and I married, I was the kind of person who would
walk a long way to avoid pain of the physical kind. Watching this
race, he was trying to understand my newfound love of racing.
There were so many things that seemed unpleasant.

For one thing, Utah Half's swim is in Utah Lake, and the mos-
quitoes in August are brutal. I had about twenty bites in the first
five minutes. The water was even slimier than usual, and I was
nervous about the fact that the first Ironman in Utah had ended
with the swim being canceled and a man dying because the waves
in Utah Lake were so bad. But I managed to make it through the
swim well enough.

Matt got to watch me stumble out of the lake as I often do. I
fell twice on the slippery boat dock. The transition from being

horizontal in the water to suddenly being upright and trying to run can be funny. At the same time, I was trying to get out of my wetsuit, which can be frustrating because it takes so long, and it feels like everyone is getting ahead of me. Then I ended up heading out on the bike with my goggles and cap still on instead of my helmet. I had to go back and do it right a second time, losing more time and getting more frustrated.

By the time Matt saw me again after the bike, the temperatures were in the 90s and I was pretty seriously dehydrated. I was so nauseated for most of the race that I could hardly walk, let alone run. I was not a happy camper, and when he saw me pass and cheered me on, I'm sure I looked terrible. Finally at the finish line, I collapsed and he tried to get me to drink and eat something while I complained that I felt like I was going to die. It didn't seem like ideal circumstances to inspire someone to want to compete in a race himself. But somehow it did.

While I ate and recovered, all Matt could talk about was how awesome the whole race had been and how much he wanted to do it the next year. He had *never* talked about wanting to do a triathlon before. He had done a half marathon that year, but triathlon seemed too complicated to him and too long. But the insanity had hit him, and more than that, it seemed possible to him. He had seen me training up close and in person for three years and he knew that I wasn't some especially talented athlete to begin with. Anyone in average health who follows a training plan can do a triathlon. I'm not saying you'll win, but you can finish, and that was all Matt wanted to do. That, and feel the love for the sport that he saw on my face as I competed.

Me, the Expert

All the way back to pick up the kids, Matt talked about what he would need to do to get ready for this race next year. He needed to do an Olympic distance triathlon first, I told him. That was what I'd done first, and I thought it was a good idea. He'd also need a new bike for himself, since his other bikes weren't suitable for triathlon racing. He'd need triathlon gear, a wetsuit, biking sunglasses, a new helmet, new running shoes and socks, a racing belt and water belt, and on and on. Matt liked lists, so it was fun to create one with him.

The next week, I made Matt a training plan which he followed religiously. One of the things I loved about this was that suddenly, I was the expert. There is nothing so intoxicating as being considered the expert by someone else. Matt is the expert at our house in all things computer related. Even though I'm the one with the father who taught computer science at a university, Matt is the one who keeps up on every new development and has figured out how to make his degree in physics into a career in computers with physics instrumentation.

In triathlon, I was now the one to listen to. I loved how this changed the kids' view of me as well. Instead of being the crazy mom who did races, I was now the person to talk to about how to get better at something. Matt modeled that admiration and the kids ran with it. I led the way to triathlon, but if it hadn't been for Matt's interest catching fire, I don't know that my kids would ever have done a single triathlon race. He knows how to make it fun far better than I do. I just know how to do it right, how to do it hard, how to make sure you finish, and how to get the right gear. The kids even talked about putting together a relay team to do the Utah Half since then, and in 2012, they did it. Faith did the swim, and was the youngest at twelve to be in the race. Sam did the bike in a respectable time, close to Matt's. And Sage suffered through the 13.5 mile run (it was a little long that year). I had the distinct pleasure of announcing them cross the finish line together. The picture of the five of us together with our medals is one of the most important pictures in our family life.

Hire a Coach or Find a Community

I hired a coach to help me through my first Ironman because I really had no idea how to do it. But Matt has relied on me as his free coach. I have the practical knowledge, but I also have the knowledge from the inside, as a racer. I know how it feels to ride for eight hours and then get off and start a marathon. I know the mistakes I've made and how to help him avoid them. I know what people say is the truth and how much of it to believe. I also know him intimately and know that sometimes work or the needs of the family have to take priority, and I can help him with a plan to work around family vacations or trips.

If you don't have someone around you who can help you chat about the details of your racing, think about finding an online community. Active.com can help you get started with chat rooms, and you can also find people through the magazines of the different sports. I recommend *Runner's World* as a magazine that has great hints and great writing about the running life. They have an online version where you can talk to people and get training plans for free. *Bicycling* is a magazine we love, even though it's fairly hard core. *Triathlete* magazine is great. There is also *Lava*, which is focused on Ironman.

If you go to a race, you can find other racers in your area and figure out when they do group rides or have group outdoor swims. There are some really experienced people there who are happy to give you advice. Listen to them. They know what they are talking about. Don't be afraid to ask questions about your specific needs. It's great to have a community of people with you at a race—people to chat with before or after and people to cheer you on even if you're the last person to finish.

The Couple Who Trains Together Can Deal with Pain Together

After Mercy's death in 2005, Matt and I had a lot of tough years. I think people who watched us from the outside thought that we handled a terrible thing like that pretty well. Maybe we did. But from the inside, it wasn't as easy as it may have looked. I was so focused on keeping myself going and working on one very specific daily goal to keep moving forward instead of looking back that I did not spend a lot of really great one-on-one time with my husband. When we talked about the baby's loss, there was so much pain involved that it was hard to speak at all. I struggled not to blame Matt for what I thought were his mistakes. I think he could feel that, even if I didn't say it out loud. And as I struggled, I lost faith in our religion more and more and that made it even more difficult for us to talk.

We had five kids together, and that was a good thing. We talked about the kids and that kept us working toward the same goals. We both wanted the best for them and we have very similar parenting styles. We struggled as Sam turned into a teenager and I threw up my hands a few times and asked Matt to take over since Sam was getting bigger and would not listen to me. When Sage started having problems with teachers at school, we talked that over and dealt with it as a couple. When Hope needed a car, we figured out how to budget it the way we have always budgeted cars—with cash.

But there were fewer date nights spent together, and less said even when we did go out. Then Matt decided to do the Utah Half and I started to train him; there was a real change in our marriage. We spent many long hours talking about triathlon and I felt a new respect, admiration, and understanding from Matt. Sometimes when I am talking to people who don't know Matt they will ask how Matt handles the fact that his wife beats him at nearly every race. Wouldn't that hurt his masculinity? Wouldn't he want to prove he was better than me? I get this response from men as well as women. I smile and say they don't know Matt. He is not interested in that kind of masculine identity.

Triathlon has allowed us to do some great things together, and not just races. Matt and I can sit and talk about geeky stuff like aero helmets for hours on end. We can talk about proper positions on bike, the best bike saddles for Ironman, heart rates, anaerobic thresholds, and on and on. We watch the World Championships for Ironman together. I keep him up to date on what events I care about and he does the same. He volunteers at my race and I volunteer at his races. Or we do races together, and with the kids. Triathlon has become a place for us to come together, and I suppose I could argue that it saved our marriage. Maybe we would have figured out another way to save it, but this is what worked for us.

Getting Prepared: Triathlon Gear, Training Bricks, and Dealing with Nerves

Gear: In Order to Do a triathlon, You MUST Have:

- A good sports bra (for women of course)
- A swimsuit
- Swim goggles
- Running shoes
- A bike
- Helmet
- Sunscreen

I put sports bra at the top because so many women think they can get away with a regular bra while running, or they make do with a lousy sports bra they've had for years. Please don't do this, especially if you wear anything above an A-cup. I spent years hating running because I didn't realize I needed a better bra. It hurts to have your boobs flapping around. It really does. Sorry guys for being so blunt about this here. Go to a good sports store and expect to spend nearly eighty dollars for a good sports bra. If you are larger and your local sports store doesn't have a size that fits you, go to www.titlenine.com. They have larger sizes and other great stuff. And whatever you do, don't wear cotton. It's horrible. Anything that has any cotton in it will make your sports life miserable.

You can spend as much on a bike as you would on a car. The more you spend, the nicer your bike. An entry level tri bike will cost around one to two thousand dollars. You can certainly use a road bike in a tri, and you probably should if you are beginning. I didn't buy a tri bike until I'd been doing triathlon for two years. You can rent bikes for a few days at a shop, too, if you want one for a specific race.

You must wear a helmet to do any racing in triathlon. Just wear the helmet anytime you are on your bike, no matter what the law in your area is. It's just stupid not to. I don't know any tri-athletes or cyclists who have not crashed at one point or another. The helmet is the only thing protecting your head, and that is your most important asset in a triathlon and in life.

Also, wear sunscreen for safety and for comfort. Get a spray on bottle of the 70 SPF and put it with your triathlon gear. I apply it after I have put on my tri suit or swim suit, but before I put on my wetsuit. If you are going to be body marked at a race, you may need to wait to apply the sunscreen until after, depending on what the race officials want. If you apply sunscreen after, be careful not to smear you numbers. Wear sunscreen whenever you are going to be outside for more than an hour.

More Advanced Triathlon Gear That Is NICE to Have:

* Wetsuit
* Bike shoes and clipless biking pedals
* Swim cap
* Nice sports socks
* Sports sunglasses
* Biking gloves
* GU packets or other brand sports gels (essentially concentrated Gatorade with sugar and electrolytes—use with water so you don't get stomach cramps)

- Gatorade
- BodyGlide
- A nice saddle

When I was first training for Ironman, I would come home with swollen eyes and be unable to see properly for hours afterward. I tried wearing regular sunglasses. They didn't help at all. I finally figured out that I had to have biking sunglasses to protect my eyes from the wind on a bike and from the debris that inevitably flies into them, especially on a six or eight hour ride.

I like GU the best, but there are other brands of sports gels like Hammergel, which is a little thinner. They are all about the consistency of honey and come in little packets or in larger containers that you can use for longer rides. The point is keeping you fueled for extensive training, longer than an hour. Some people use GU packets and Gatorade. Some people use GU packets and only water. See what works for you by trying it out in training. One thing I should note is that after I trained for my most recent Ironman, the hygienist at the dentist's office complained that I had significantly more plaque on my teeth than on other visits. She recommended switching out Gatorade with water at least a couple times during long rides to protect my teeth.

BodyGlide is the brand name for a sports-specific, anti-chafing lubricant. I like it the best of the ones I've tried, but you may have a different experience. The key is not to use Vaseline, as petroleum products can damage your wetsuit material. Some people I know simply use PAM spray, which doesn't hurt wetsuits, but certainly seems strange to spray all over yourself. It's cheap, though. The key is that it needs to not wash off in the water, so it will help you slip out of the wetsuit when the swim is over.

Matt and I both had the experience of using a standard bike shop saddle while we were training for Ironman and discovering that we had extensive crotch pain that didn't go away for days. People would tell me I would just get used to it, but I didn't seem to be getting used to it at all. Finally, after some research online, I went and bought a CRMO brand saddle with a hole in the middle called a "butterfly." Matt got a male version and both of us immediately stopped having the pain. There are lots of brands now that use the same strategy of cutting out the middle of the saddle and making sure it is still stable with strong materials elsewhere. If you have crotch pain while biking, try one out. Yes, you have to get your butt used to long rides and there is some toughening up to be done. But a new saddle may be in order.

Bricks

Bricks are the triathlon term for workouts that are back-to-back with different disciplines. Most typically, triathletes will do a swim-bike brick or a bike-run brick, because those are the two that will be done in a race. Sometimes, a reverse triathlon will require a run-bike brick or a bike-swim brick, just to confuse you. I have found that I do almost all of my workouts as bricks of one kind or another. Usually, I do a bike-run brick, because I find it comfortable to warm up on the bike and then move to a challenging run. These are the standard bricks, but there are lots of other choices for bricks.

A beginning triathlete will want to practice whatever transitions are particular to the race ahead, but otherwise, transitions of any kind are good for you. I find that I have to work harder to swim if I've done weight lifting and bike or elliptical first, and that is sometimes a good thing. If I swim first and then do weights, I can't lift as much, but I just target weights one rung below my normal and still get a good workout.

Of course, you want to get your body used to being able to go from swimming horizontally to running and biking, but ideally, you should train your body so that it can handle anything you throw at it. You also want to train yourself to realize what works and what doesn't work for you.

One of the workouts I do now and again is a continual brick. I will bike for ten minutes, then hop off the bike and run a mile, then back on the bike again, over and over again. You can make these intervals longer, thirty minutes on the bike, two or three miles of running. This is easy for me since I'm indoors on my own equipment. But it's also great for when the kids want to work out with me. They can use either the bike or the treadmill that I'm not using, and they can still be with me and talk to me.

How to Deal with Nerves

Everyone gets nervous before a race. Some people are more affected the night before. Others get sick right before the race begins. Feeling nauseated, dizzy, like you are an idiot, like this is impossible—all perfectly normal.

Nerves Are Part of Your Body's Preparation

I have begun to believe that these nerves are actually part of your body's physical preparation for a race, and that they are important, even necessary. When I feel that racing heart beat that makes it hard to sleep, I remind myself that this is my body getting me energized. Nerves are just energy and you can direct that energy in the direction you want it to go.

Visualize the Race Course

The night before a race (or sometimes a few days before the race), I will start to visualize the race as much as possible. If I've done that race before, this is easy because I know the tricky turns the race takes. I know where the turnaround point is for the bike. I know what times I am hoping for. I try to imagine myself on the bike, the motion in my legs feeling smooth and free. I try to imagine getting into the water and how it will feel to start stroking when the gun goes off. I try to imagine the other racers, some faster than me, some not. There is a wonderful feeling, being in a race with other people. You have a community right there, cheering for you even if they don't say a word. They're with you.

Visualize the Finish Line

I also try to imagine what it will feel like to cross the finish line. I try to tell myself that no matter what has happened in the race, I will feel good about myself at the finish line. I have had bad races, believe me. I've had races where I crashed in the race and had to get up, bloody and bruised, get back on the bike, finish the bike, and still do the run. I've had races where I was the one who caused the crash and hurt someone else, and I apologized and moved on. I've had races where someone else hurt me, and I've had to move on. I've had races where I had to start walking, where I felt like I wasn't going to finish, but I did. There are a lot of things that can happen in a race, good and bad. I think it's good to know that when you're preparing mentally. Then you aren't surprised when it happens. You know how to fix a bike flat. You know what to do if you feel like you can't go on. You have a plan, try walking for a few minutes, then try to run again. Try drinking some water after you've thrown up. See if you can hold it down. And continue to see the finish and you running through it.

Make Lists

Matt makes lists. He writes down everything he needs to bring to the race, everything he needs to get done before the race, then checks them off one by one, so he feels ready. Perhaps he is the list making expert in the family. It is his way of dealing with his nerves.

Know Your Mantra

I have rhythmic mantras I say to myself during the swim, the bike, and the run. These will sound stupid, but I say "You can do it,

Mette" and "Pain feels good." I also count to keep myself focused on my body's motions and not other things that can distract me. When I am swimming, instead of thinking about the gross things in the water or the fish that might touch me, I focus on my stroke, on what I can control.

Helping Kids with Nerves

If you have kids doing a race with you, your job is to help them deal with their nerves. Keep them focused on the moment. Give them something to do, like setting up their own gear. Guide them through it, but don't do it for them. Then talk them through each part of the race as you think about it yourself. Tell them you know they can do it. Also tell them that if they just do their best, you will be proud of them. Remind them of the rules on the bike about how far back to stay (three bike lengths). Remind them always to pass on the left, and to let others pass them on the left by staying right. Remind them to be aware of cars if it is an open course. Your positive focus will help to keep them calm and ready.

Focus on the Positive

Try to think of things in a positive light rather than a negative one. Everything is part of the experience. If you have a problem, all that means is that you probably won't have that problem again. You will have learned how to deal with it. A problem does not mean it's the end of the race. Be flexible and accept that this is not going to go perfectly. Races do not go perfectly for anyone. The people who do well are the people who have done it often enough that they know how to deal with problems. Problems aren't the enemy. They are a chance for you to learn something. I mean this.

Celebrate

One other thing I would recommend to deal with nerves is to celebrate. Celebrate that you signed up for the race by going out the night before. Buy yourself something to use in the race as a prize. And celebrate afterward, no matter how the race goes, celebrate that you signed up and that you attempted it. Have something to look forward to as you are racing, or if you are doing it with kids, have something waiting for them to look forward to. Not a surprise, something they *know* is coming. Tell your kids or yourself that you are proud. Buy yourself a medal if you care about that. Wear your T-shirt all day. Tell people what you did. Remind yourself what you did. *Celebrate!*

CHAPTER 10

IT'S NOT ALL SUNSHINE AND ROSES

A s a writer, I have failed a lot. I often remind students when I visit classrooms that I wrote twenty (really bad) novels before I wrote one that sold. I've met a lot of other writers who tell people that the first novel never sells—and sometimes not the second or third. But I have never met anyone who wrote twenty novels before being published. This is probably proof that I am not naturally gifted as a writer, but I do not believe much in talent anyway. I believe in persistence, and I was very persistent before I was published.

Looking at Failure as a Path to Success

No one wants to fail. But being afraid of failure makes it difficult to be successful, Failure often happens along the way to success. At least, that's the way I think about it.

I failed as a high school swimmer. I completely gave up any idea that I was athletic until I was in my thirties. But once I started doing triathlon, I had a lot of success. Sure, there were races that did not work out. I made many mistakes as I was learning. In one of my early races, I didn't have a road bike, so tried to rent one, but got to the shop too late the night before. I had to use the mountain bike I had at home and that made me really slow. I think I was the very last person to finish the bike distance in that race. But I kept going and I made up time a little more in the run. I loved that race and it made me stronger.

I've had races where I injured myself either during the race itself or before the race, so I couldn't go at full speed. I've also had races with a flat tire or two flat tires that made me lose time. I've been stupid enough to lose time because I put my helmet on backward and the volunteers had to stop me before I got out of transition. And of course, I've had races where I simply didn't feel my best.

The important thing is to keep trying. If I am bleeding from a crash, or if I am confused and end up doing extra distance on the bike (or the swim or run), I keep going. I finish what I start. If I pay for a race, I do it. I give my all to it. I want my kids to see me do this. I want to be proud of myself enough not to quit, even if I am the very last competitor across the finish line.

If you live and race like this, failure is never failure. A bad race is just one to tell stories about. And that is true in life, too. You can always learn a lesson from a failure, and that makes it not a failure at all, but a stopping place along the path to success. There are ways to succeed even while failing, just succeeding in a different way than the one you expected. And sometimes failure makes you realize a truth that you did not see before, and that can be a kind of success, too.

Crash and Recovery

If you are a Tour de France aficionado, you have surely watched the reel of bike crashes that gets ever longer as the years go on. The fun ones are the ones when you know the people in the crash got back up as soon as they could, and continued biking. Most of the time, it is more like Dominoes, one guy crashes and then everyone behind him crashes. Sometimes a mechanical failure starts the collision. More often, it is a result of someone missing a sharp turn, or the weather plays a factor. It is July, and you would think—hot and dry, but in Europe, July can also mean torrential rainfall, and that is no good for the slick tires that professional cyclists use. One slip and you're down and out, and maybe, a bunch of other cyclists on your team are out, too.

No professional cyclist has avoided crashes. They all have stories to tell of crashes in training and out. It is part of the life. A broken collarbone is like a badge of honor. You will get five or six of those over the course of your career. "Road rash" as it's called when you scrape off your jersey or shorts and then a good deal of skin beneath, and the blood drips down your leg as you get back on your bike, is generally considered nothing to worry about. Wearing a helmet these days is required. If it were not, I suspect many racers would still be going without helmets, just to prove how tough they are.

Matt and I have often thought that Cervélos, one of the bikes advertised on the Tour de France and ridden by a lot of professionals, are the best looking and fastest bikes around. So, when I got a nice check for selling a book, I decided on a new Cervélo P2 with nice wheels. I should have expected that I would end up in a bike crash sooner rather than later. But, when it happened only a few weeks after I bought my new baby—well, I am not sure if I was more upset about what happened to me or to my bike.

I took it out late in the season on a Saturday planning to do a ninety-mile ride on the Legacy Parkway. There are no cars, and it's safer and less noisy to ride on. I didn't count on the rain. In August in Utah we don't get a lot of rain, but about half way through my ride the rain started. It wasn't a downpour and I didn't think the trail was particularly slick. Honestly, I was more afraid of the mosquitos that would come with the rain than I was of the slick roads. There is a very sharp right hand turn at about mile eight on Legacy. I slowed to take it, but I did not slow enough. One moment I was thinking, I am going to be fine. The next moment, I was on the pavement. It happened that fast.

I don't really remember hitting the ground. I just remember the pain of being on the ground and deciding that I wasn't quite ready to get up. I am not sure how much time passed exactly, but my next coherent thought was that I wanted to turn off my timer on my watch so that I didn't mess up my data. That probably says way too much about my personality and the importance of data to me.

A minute or so later, an older woman on a leisure bike came up behind me. I'd passed her a few minutes back, blown past her in fact. She came up and saw me lying on the ground, got off her bike (I'm sure she wasn't thinking to herself how stupid I was, and how this was the just deserts of someone who was riding so hard) and bent over to help me. She asked me if I needed her to call someone. But I knew I hadn't broken any bones. I was in pain, but it was just road rash. Bradley Wiggins would just get back on the bike and keep going, dealing with it on the road or at the end of the race.

So that was what I did. I told the woman thanks, and she went on her way. Then I took a look at my wounds. I had fallen on my right side, and my shorts had been pulled way up so that my entire right thigh was raw and bleeding. Worse, my right arm from my wrist to my elbow was bleeding badly, especially right at the elbow. The back of my right hand was hurt too, although I had been wearing fingerless gloves, so mostly it was just the top half of each finger that had skin torn off. I couldn't imagine really what a doctor would do except bandage me up and send me home. And, well, I still had a workout I wanted to finish.

So I pulled my shorts back over my bleeding leg. My arm stung badly as I pressed it into the aero pads on the bike, which were salty with sweat and everyone knows how good that feels in an open wound. I rode another forty miles after the bike crash at a twenty-one mile per hour pace. Finally, I biked home on Highway 89 and put my bike into the garage. I had to take one of the kids to a birthday party and I was running a little late, so I threw on some sweats over the road rash, and ran a comb through my hair. I picked out a book from my collection—an autographed one—put it into a gift bag for the birthday child and headed out the door with child in tow.

After the birthday drop off, I drove home and faced my injuries. I got into the bathtub and hissed through my teeth at the pain of water on my arms and legs. I washed up as best I could, and got out. Matt arrived home from a long run just in time to see the full extent of the injuries as I was trying to decide what to put on—cover the wounds fully or not?

He went out immediately to the local drug store and spent thirty dollars on wound care supplies, including giant bandage pads. He also bought a disinfectant that promised it would numb the wound. He came home, ready to spray it on. I lay down in the bathroom for medic Matt. At this point, the kids were aware something was wrong, so they came up to watch. I figured it was good for them to see the effects of my error, and to watch Matt taking care of the wounds. So Sage and Hope were right there as Matt sprayed on the disinfectant.

I was not expecting it to hurt at all (that was the whole point, after all, to make it feel better), and so I screamed when it went on. Matt realized afterward that the spray had alcohol in it and was not meant for open wounds. It burned for a long time, but at least the wound was clean. Matt smeared me up with ointment and then put on bandages. I felt like a bandage factory as I limped around the rest of that day and some of the next.

Despite the pain, I felt like I was pretty cool. It was like an initiation of sorts. Like a baptism of blood and pain. I was a real biker now. I had suffered like a real Tour de France team member. And I had kept going. I had crashed, but I took satisfaction in knowing that it did not kill me. As they say, it only made me stronger. I am still afraid of cars hitting me and don't go out often on the roads with my bike, but crashes don't frighten me the way they used to. I survived.

In 2011, I crashed during a bike race, the US TriSports Stansbury Tri in September. I was not paying attention at the place where the sprinters turn around and the Olympic racers go straight. I crashed into someone turning, and the volunteers got me right back on my bike. The brakes were stuck on for the next fifteen miles of the course, so no matter how hard I pedaled, my maximum speed with the drag was ten miles an hour. It was tiring and frustrating at once, but I finished the course and went back out on the run, still bleeding. When I crossed the finish line, I grabbed a water bottle and headed over to the medical tent to get some wound care. The guy I had crashed into was there, and I apologized to him for causing the crash. I think I got the worst of it, but I still felt bad.

I won third place in my age group for that race even with the crash, so I have a medal as well as a fine scar on my left elbow to remember that race. Scars are better than medals in my opinion, to tell a story about pain. Pain is a natural part of life. You are not going to avoid it. I do not invite it, but I am not afraid of it either. After crashing on my bike, I felt pain every step of that 10k run, but it didn't stop me. You just keep going, gritting your teeth against it. You get stronger, and you know that nothing can stop you after that.

Finding the Success in Failure

Crashing and getting back up is something to be proud of, but DNFing (did not finish) at a race is something that no athlete ever brags about. I have only DNF'd once in my life of triathlon, but that race is one that in some ways defines me, both as a person and as an athlete. I have never gone back and done the race again, though I certainly feel the need to at some point, to erase the black mark of the DNF off my memory. For now, I have to live with it, and I think it is important to talk about it now and again. This was a real failure, but there are ways in which I managed to turn it into a success, and for that, I am proud of myself.

The race was LOTOJA, an annual bike race that goes 206 miles from Logan, Utah to Jackson Hole, Wyoming each September. It is the longest single day bike race in the country and it crosses three states, ending in the beautiful Tetons. LOTOJA is so popular that they have a lottery entry. I was lucky enough to get in on my first try. I thought it would be an interesting challenge, after Ironman, more about finishing the distance than about my time.

It seemed like they had a reasonable time limit set up. You could bike essentially all day, at a little less than fifteen miles per hour and finish before the cut off, which was simply when it was too dark to be safe. The bike has always been my strongest leg of triathlon, so I was eager to try out an all bike race. I have done running races, everything from 5k to half marathon and marathon to ultramarathons. I have done swimming races as an adult, too, where I've had to remember how to dive from the blocks into the water without looking like an idiot (that's the height of my expectations). But I had never done a bike race, so this was my new challenge.

It sounds good on paper, doesn't it? Maybe I was made to be a biker. I had great hopes and dreams before the race started. The only problem is—I am by nature a very solitary athlete. I like the competition in races. I just don't like it on a regular basis. The coach I hired to get me through my first Ironman thought this was one of the strangest things about me. He kept telling me which long bikes I was "allowed" to do with other riders and which ones I "had" to do alone. I did all of them alone because I don't mind spending six to eight hours by myself. I like the time to think and just feel the quiet of the world around me. As a mother of five kids, believe me, there is plenty of noise and chaos inside my house on a regular basis.

But cycling is a team sport in a way I did not really understand when I signed up for this race. In triathlon, there are all these rules about how close you can be to another bike and how long you can remain in a drafting position (fifteen seconds) without being disqualified. But LOTOJA is all about drafting, finding the right group, and being with a group the whole way. Only the last little bit of the race do people begin to peel off the group and try to win as an individual (not that I ever saw that part—but I have heard about it).

I just kept training for LOTOJA as if it were a really long bike section of a triathlon. I trained indoors almost all the time. I trained alone. This was a big mistake. I didn't find a group ride to join, though my local bike store sponsors them every Saturday. I didn't want to have to worry about being social while I was working out. It's always been one of my weakest points, that social aspect of my life. I can be social. It just takes effort, and that is hard to do when I am also biking. Those are excuses, I know, but I let myself use them.

I also had an equipment problem. It turns out my very expensive Cervélo is considered a time trial (TT) bike and not allowed on LOTOJA or other drafting races. If your hands are on aerobars, you can't break as fast, and you can hurt a long line of people. So I had to figure out another bike to ride. I put off this problem until the last moment and rented a road bike for a few days just before the race. I somehow expected that it would be good enough for me to ride it a few times even though the race itself was going to be more than twelve hours.

My last problem was that I could not fall asleep the night before the race. This was a frequent problem for me before races at the time. I had terrible insomnia and had gone to the doctor to get a prescription for Ambien. But even taking two pills of Ambien did not keep me from tossing and turning until 2:00 a.m. I had to be up at 5:30 a.m., and this was not a good amount of sleep to race on.

These were all mistakes, and if you stick around runners or other adult athletes long enough, you may tire of hearing about all the reasons that a particular race did not go well for them. On one hand, this can be annoying. It was a bad race, end of story, right? Get over it. But on the other hand, one of the reasons we are drawn to racing is the belief that we have that we can figure it out, triumph over our problems, and have the perfect race. It doesn't happen often, that perfect race, but it does happen now and again, and I think we are always hoping for it to happen again.

The plan for this race was to get the kids up early and throw them into the van with my bike. They could sleep until we got up to the starting line. Then Matt would drive around and be my support vehicle (a requirement of this race). He would meet me at specific locations along the course and give me food and emotional support. Then he would be there at the finish line up in Wyoming, and we would crash at a hotel before heading back to Utah the next day.

I've figured out some of the mistakes I made, but I'm not sure any of them explain the feeling I had in the first twenty minutes of the race. My heart rate was sky high for the pace I was hitting, and I felt horrible. It may have simply been a bad day. You can never know for sure because you can never replay everything again with just one thing changed. I do remember the quaint, small town of Logan, pressed up against the Wasatch Mountains. We headed west at first, away from the mountains into the flats around the Great Salt Lake. It was September, and the colors were brown and gold and red. It should have felt great. I should have been feeling like this was easy. The beginning of a race should never be hard. But it was.

I was dropped early by the group I started with, though one nice woman tried to stay with me and help me along by letting me draft off her. She gave up after about an hour and I was on my own. I thought that if I just kept going I would be able to finish at least, even if I didn't do well. I suspect I was not eating or drinking enough, but again, it is hard to know how much of an effect that had on me. It might have been no more than a bad day.

I hit Idaho and the big climbs began. I wish that I had been enjoying the race more and could have seen the beauty of the course. We were on these tiny roads, hardly a car in sight, and it was late September, the perfect time to see the change in the leaves, spectacular in the Rockies. But my focus was on the blacktop in front of me, and keeping my pedals moving. I found myself with a small group of the slowest people. We worked our way up and then up again, following switchback after switchback. I was miserable. I began to think about the possibility of not finishing this race.

After hours of climbing and feeling discouraged, I got to the top of the final hill in the first section of the course. At that point, I knew that I had about twenty miles of straight downhill, which is essentially rest on the bike. It should have been a moment of triumph. Here the trees were so close together that they were almost shaking hands over the roads. I could see leaves swirling all around me, even with my head down. I felt cushioned from the sounds of the world by the forest around me. Maybe I could still do this, I thought. Get some food in, get some rest, and I could finish if I just kept going.

But it was not to be. At the final feed station at the top of the hill, I got off my bike to eat and drink a little. When I tried to get back on, I started in too high a gear, and could not turn the wheel over. Without thinking I just kept trying to turn the wheel instead of stepping off; I fell over and hit my right shoulder hard. It was the last straw, the last proof that something was terribly wrong at this race. One of the volunteers ran over and helped push me a bit to get me started, but the race was over for me at that point. I pedaled miserably downhill through incredible scenery, but I could only think about the race being over.

I met Matt and the kids at the halfway point and told him I was done. I think he didn't know if he should tell me to keep going or not. I told him flatly I didn't want encouragement. I wanted him to figure out what to do to get me out of the race and take me home. He found the right official to check me out of the race and basically make sure they weren't looking for me along the road. Then I got into the car. I was in so much pain that it was really hard to identify which part of my body it was coming from. In the end, it didn't make sense for us to just go home since we'd already paid for a hotel room and the kids had been looking forward to a vacation.

So we kept going to the finish line, passing the bikers who were ahead of me. This was a rather painful part of the trip, watching those who were doing what I had not been able to. But somehow, I was able to focus on my kids and tell them a story. It's one of our family traditions that on a vacation, while we are on the long drive, I will tell an all original story to my kids. I don't think up these stories beforehand. They are truly spur-of-the-moment, and they are just for my kids, no desire for publication. On this particular occasion, I told a long story about a kid who found a door into another world in which there were creatures called "Kibbers" who were as big as elephants but you could ride on them. I don't remember much of the story beyond that, but the kids remember it well and frequently ask me to tell it again, which I cannot do for the life of me.

As we drove, we caught a glimpse of the beautiful Tetons at sunset, the pillars of gold and red streaked with light. It would have been a great moment to be at the end of the ride, but we turned away from the finish and headed west to our hotel. I tried my best to hide my pain and act cheerful, as if this were any other family vacation. Once we arrived at the hotel, to my surprise, we had a great time. Sam was excited because there was a mini kitchen and he could cook some food, including a banana glazed in Gatorade left over from my race food. There was also a pool. We went to the pool, and I tried to play with the kids like Matt did, even agreeing to play chicken with Sam on my shoulders.

This was when I discovered the result of the fall on my right shoulder. The pain of Sam's weight on my shoulders was excruciating. I cried out in pain and threw him off, then sat gasping. It was months before this pain went away. I couldn't swim during this time because of the pain in my shoulder. I self-diagnosed it, as I often do with my injuries. Like many other injuries, this one needed mostly rest and patience, which I tried to give it.

Looking back on this failed race, I am proud of myself even so. I wish I had not made the mistakes I had. I still want to go back to do this race again and conquer it. But in the face of my own disappointment, I did not let my kids down. We had one of the best family vacations in their memory and that is still something that I cherish. Most of our family vacations these days are related to some race that either Matt, or I, or the kids are doing. As important to me as a race is, with all the preparation and expectations that I put into it, my kids are more important. I feel like I showed them that in September of 2007. In the midst of failure as an athlete, I succeeded as a parent, and that is the more important race.

You Are Not Your Time

Speaking of failures, there are more where that came from, though of a slightly different flavor. In the spring of 2008, I trained hard for the Ogden Marathon in hopes of getting a PR (personal record) and qualifying for the Boston Marathon, which is every runner's dream. In hopes of achieving this dream, I had given up most of my triathlon training. I slavishly followed an advanced training plan on The Runner's World website (www.runnersworld.com). There was one day a week where I did killer intervals, doing quarter-mile, half-mile, and full-mile sprints at a six-minute pace. One day a week I did a tempo pace run, which is supposed to be at race pace, but not as long as the race. I think I hated the tempo runs the most. There were also the long run days, which I did not do at the pace recommended in the plan. I did them harder because I figured that would get me more ready for the race.

Yeah, here's the analysis part again: I shouldn't have done more than the plan recommended. I was anxious to prove to myself that I was getting faster and that I could hit the pace I wanted to reach for the race. That meant that when I had an eighteen mile run that was supposed to be at nine minutes per mile, I ran it at 7:45 because that was my goal pace. You can imagine that this led to me being rather fatigued, especially since I did a long run at goal pace every week, along with the intervals and tempo running. I was forcing my body to hit race pace every week, but not giving it any recovery or taper time as you would in a race. Stupid, stupid, stupid! And I thought this would lead to good results? Well, it didn't, as I'm sure you already guessed.

When I was working with my coach for Ironman training and showed him my logs for the past four months, the first thing he had me do was take three days completely off, plus a weekend. I was not *allowed* to do any training. I had to do some serious recovery before he could ramp me up to the insane level he had planned for me. My point here is that a lot of people actually sabotage their efforts by not resting enough. While you are resting, your muscles actually get stronger. You tear them up while training, and that makes you weaker. It is when you make sure to get in enough protein,vitamins, and minerals in, and you rest and let your body rebuild those muscles stronger than they were before (better, stronger, faster—yes, I saw *The Million Dollar Man* when I was a kid, too), that you become a better athlete. Tearing yourself up every week may prove that you can deal with more pain than other people do, but it doesn't actually make you stronger.

After three months of killing myself like this, I went out and did a 30k race that was meant to be a tune-up. Instead, I went out too fast and ended up walking toward the end. And 30k is only 18.6 miles. It's not anywhere near a full marathon. I had done all my racing in training and now I had to take some time off. I went back to swimming and biking to try to recover, but it was too little, too late. Three weeks later, in May 2008, I toed the line with my husband and several friends to start the Ogden Marathon. I tried to push myself. But it didn't happen. I had made my mistakes, and I was going to have to suffer the consequences.

I was tired from the very first step and I knew from the first mile that I wouldn't be making my goal time of 7:30 per mile. I knew by mile three that I wouldn't even be making my back-up goal time of 7:45 per mile. At mile eight, the woman from my neighborhood I had beat by ten minutes at our last match-up passed me. At mile nine, I knew I wouldn't even make my previous PR time of 8:20 per mile. By mile ten, my sister-in-law who had claimed she only wanted to finish and had no goal time passed me. By mile thirteen, Matt passed me. Yet I continued to run. I ran past the mile 13.1 point, where I could have quit and taken a bus down to the end of the course. I was determined that I would finish this race. I was in pain and I was discouraged, but if I kept going, I could do it.

When my legs started cramping at mile nineteen, I began the slow walk down the canyon as I realized that my finishing time would probably be close to my first marathon time, when I hadn't run more than six miles in training. And yet I kept going. I was not going to DNF this time.

Men and women who seemed too overweight to be running a marathon passed me. A woman who seemed too old to be running a marathon passed me. A woman who was six inches shorter than I was (and I am very short) passed me. A man who was in the walk-run stage of his marathon passed me and looked back to ask if I was OK. I told him I was fine. I kept walking. I knew that I would finish the marathon in time to get a medal, to be an official finisher and somehow, that still mattered to me. I got more and more nauseated as I went, but still, I kept going.

I had a long time as I walked those last six miles to think about why I was still walking. Yes, in some ways, I was able to enjoy the magnificent scenery of the race more. I had a long time to stare at the lush trees of spring in the Utah desert, the beautiful waterfall over the precipice down to the river.

Spectators called out encouragement. "Good job," they called to me. "You're almost there. Keep going," they said. I smiled and waved back at them, embarrassed that they felt obliged to share their energy for me, who was beyond help. I began to cross people who had finished and were coming back to encourage their friends on. And I realized that I had finally found the reason that I kept going. You see, I had come to the end of myself and I found that my race time didn't matter anymore.

This wasn't about having a time to brag about anymore. This was about being stripped down to the bones and seeing that even if I wasn't an athlete, even if I never raced again, I was still me underneath all my times and accomplishments. And that me was someone I was proud to be. That me was someone who kept going when she could keep going, even when her dream times had passed her by. Even when she was embarrassed, she kept going.

When I got home, I put the medal from that race in a very special place of honor and I still value it above all the other medals I've ever won. This medal is the one that reminds me of the day I came to the end of myself, and maybe, the beginning too.

Biking Tips

Buying Your Biking Gear

In order to do anything other than a basic finish-the-course race in triathlon, you will need to become familiar with your local specialty bike shop. This can be intimidating. Everyone there knows the lingo. They wear weird clothes and they all seem to know each other. You walk in, people stare at you and you have no idea what to say.

Most bike shops will have an extensive set of bikes set up along the edges of the store. These bikes are not really meant to be tried out, but you can look at them and see what you may be buying. The problem is that you probably have no idea what kind of bike you want unless you spend hours of time researching bikes in magazines beforehand. And even then, you will still want the advice of the bike experts.

Other parts of the store will include specialized bike clothing. To men in particular these outfits may seem ridiculous. There will be tight fitting tops for triathlon made almost entirely of Lycra. Then there are the even more ridiculous looking bike shorts that have what looks like a diaper of padding between your legs. And bike shorts that have built in suspenders to keep them in place. Yeah, you will want these. If you don't get good bike shorts, you will end up in serious pain. I have been doing heavy biking for a lot of years and I do not often wear bike shorts anymore, but that is because I have decided to leave the padding on my seat and have a specialized butterfly seat with a cut out center to relieve pressure. Real bikers have much harder seats and they laugh at me. You can choose between the diaper and the cushier seat.

The bike tops have tons of pockets in different places. This may look weird to you, but bikers, unlike runners, are expected to carry their own food and water during most races and training. They put water bottles on their bikes, of course, but also in the pockets in the back of their shirts. Biking tops will also have sleeves, which provide more coverage for those who will be outside in the sun for hours on end. This makes a lot of sense.

Other things you will see in a biking store include bike pumps, either in the large variety to keep at home or the small variety to put in a pack on your bike. Also you will find canisters of air to pump up your tires. Please ask for help in buying these and learning how to properly use them. Don't be one of those bikers who gets a flat and has no idea how to change it. When I was training for my Ironman, I spent three days learning how to take tires off and put them back on—back tires and front. Learn how to do this and carry your own supplies on your bike. It also helps enormously when dealing with nerves before a race to feel confident enough to handle a flat on your own.

There are a lot of things you can buy to make it possible to bike in colder weather. Wool socks, booties, and heavier waterproof coats. I admit, I do not often go out when it is cold. I do not often go outside at all. I am afraid of traffic. I tend to train indoors on a trainer with my bike, one with a video of the courses I want to ride. But if you're going outside in the winter, get the right gear. Winter or summer, you should have special biking socks. These will help you to not get blisters. There are some people who do Ironman with no socks, but I am not one of them.

A helmet is another thing you will need to buy. A good one will cost you about one hundred dollars. You don't need one of the aero helmets to start with (those are the ones that look like inverted ice cream cones and are smooth). A good helmet for everyday use will have lots of vents in it and will feel comfortable. Ask for help to get fitted for the proper helmet.

If you already have a bike, you can take it to a bike shop to get it fixed, but if it is a cheap bike that you have bought at a store like Wal-Mart, they will not want to fix it up. It will cost more to try than the bike cost new, and they still won't be able to make it right. It will frustrate the technicians. They would feel like artists being asked to paint with finger paints. They are used to more expensive materials and the proper results.

This leads me to the bike. This is the biggest purchase that you will make to do triathlon. An entry level triathlon or road bike will put you back about fifteen hundred dollars. When you enter the store, catch the eye of one of the people at the register or go to the back where there are people working on repairs. Tell them what you want and ask them for advice. They like to be asked for advice. Trust me. Most of them are not triathletes. They are cyclists. But nonetheless, there is some crossover and they will usually be willing to talk about things like aero bars and disc wheels (though those are more advanced). A road bike will work for a triathlon, and you can add on aerobars later if you want. There is some difference in the set up of a tri bike. They are designed to make it so that you can run after you get off them, using less of your hamstring muscles which you will need for running. But honestly, they are so similar it may not make any difference to you.

I can't tell you what bike you should buy. I'm not an expert. I can say that I like my Quintana Roo and I also like my Cervélo. I think that Trek is a good brand, as well. Do not stint on the components like your gear wheels and your derailleurs. You can upgrade with better wheels later if you'd like. I started with a beginner bike and then after about four years of racing, moved up to a more expensive bike. My nice Cervélo P2 cost more than most of our cars. Our kids joke around that we have to lock our cars only when our bikes are in them.

Equipment Musts

Get a proper saddle

I like butterfly seats with a cut out in the middle. Find what works for you.

Get a bike fit

This costs around two hundred dollars. It will save you pain and time in the end. A bike fit after you buy your bike will maximize your potential on your new bike. A bike consult before you buy your bike can tell you the right frame size and type to get to fit your body type.

Get an aero helmet

You really only need this if you are going to do long races like an Ironman or half Ironman.

Get bike shoes and clipless pedals

Figure out how to use them. Practice in your garage while holding on to the wall. Go in and out two dozen times before you go outside. Expect that you may have an accident and fall over. You will live.

The last thing I have to say is to keep your local bike store in business. Please do not go into your bike store, get advice there for free, and then go buy a bike online. If you do that, the bike store will go out of business, and you won't have anyone to go to for help with bike fits, advice, personal attention, or repairs.

Biking Basics

Most world class bikers have a cadence of ninety to a hundred revolutions per minute (rpm). This means if you count only your right leg hitting the bottom part of the stroke, you will count ninety to one hundred per minute. Sound familiar? It is the same as in running, when you are trying to hit ninety to one hundred foot strikes on your right leg per minute. You can buy a computer that will tell you how many revolutions you are hitting per minute or you can measure it indoors on a trainer by looking at a watch and counting for ten seconds, then multiplying by six.

•   If you are on a real course, lean forward on your aerobars or get into a proper aero position either on downhills or on flats. This helps with air resistance, which is a bigger factor the faster you go.

•   Slow **before** you get to a turn. Don't put the brakes on while you are in the turn itself. Aim to go into the turn a little wide, and come out a little wide if you have room. Speed up as you come out of the turn. If you stand, you may want to gear up.

- On hills, your cadence should be eighty revolutions per minute or lower. If you stand, you may want to gear down because you put more pressure on the pedals then. It should still be easy to turn your crank. Consider getting a different crank set if you go up hills and frequently struggle.

- The most common mistake I see with bikers is that they keep their seats too low. Your knees should only bend very slightly at the bottom of the stroke. It's possible to put your seat too high, but if you do, you will be reaching from side to side to finish your stroke.

- It's a good idea to spend a few minutes each week doing one-legged cycling. If you do this indoors, it is a lot easier. You clip out one foot and rest it on the frame of your bike, then spin hard with only one leg for one minute at a lower gear than you could probably do with both legs, then take fifteen seconds to switch legs and do the same thing over again. This will help even out some of the imbalances in your pedaling. Many people tend to use one leg more than the other (often the right). Also, many people will only push down and not finish the full stroke by pulling up. One-legged cycling forces you to do the whole stroke.

- Always carry a water bottle with you. One of my children refuses to drink Gatorade, which I think is unfortunate. Gatorade is a cheap and easy way to get some calories and it has been proven that the taste of real sugar signals to your brain that you can keep going harder for longer. At the very least, you need to drink water often.

Illness and Injuries

We All Get Sick

If you are sick, here is a guideline for deciding what you should do:

- If you have a cold and you feel "Blah," you can still do a workout, but an easier and shorter one than the one you had planned. If you are sick for one or two days, you can continue with the rest of the plan when you are well.
- If you are having your period, ladies, you can probably still do a workout, but just make it easier and shorter.
- If you feel "off" for some unknown reason and don't end up showing any signs of illness, just shrug and don't worry about it. Everyone has bad days that they can't explain. It's likely just a bad day. It doesn't mean that you are never going to be able to do the race or that you won't be able to get your PR (personal record).
- If you have a fever, do not workout. Stay in bed and take it easy. Give yourself one more full day to recover after your fever is completely gone.
- If you are throwing up and can't keep anything down, don't do a workout. Do an easy one the next day.
- If you are sick for three or more days, do not continue with your current training plan. You will need to go back a week and redo that week's workouts before you can step up to the next week.
- If you are sick for more than a week, you will probably have to start at the beginning of your training plan again. I know this feels discouraging, but it will be more discouraging to try to do something that your body is not prepared for.

Injuries Happen to the Best of Us

If you are suffering an injury of any kind, my first advice is to leave it alone. Don't do anything that makes it hurt. If you can stand to just stay off it, that is your best first choice. If it hurts even when you aren't using it, it is probably time to see a doctor.

If you are injured in some visible way, like from a fall on your bike or while running, the best advice is RICE (rest, ice, compress, elevate). The more swelling you see, the more your body is trying to heal a specific wounded area.

Many injuries are caused by increasing training volume too quickly. A general rule of thumb is no more than 10% per week. You can also push yourself too hard, even if you aren't increasing training distance or time too much. If you spend more than twenty percent of your training doing sprint work, you could also end up with injuries. If you overdo it, you will have to step back and rest for a few weeks before you start again, and you may have to go more slowly the second time around.

Other injuries can be caused by poor equipment. In particular, the wrong pair of running shoes can be disastrous. If you have knee problems, shin splints, or hip pain, and you either have old shoes or a pair of brand new ones, consider the possibility that you simply need to invest in new shoes. A consult at a running store will cost about as much as one visit to the doctor and may do more.

Then there are problems related to flexibility, for which I advise you to avoid icing completely. In fact, more heat may be called for, to help your muscles warm up before you stretch.

Here are some common injuries that need more then RICE:

IT Band

When I did my first marathon with very little training, I was in a tremendous amount of pain. I couldn't run for months afterward without pain in my knees that radiated up to my hip. I figured out at some point that this was called the IT Band or Iliotibial band syndrome. There are a lot of exercises and stretches you can find online to help with this. The easiest one I did was to cross my legs and lean forward, trying to touch my toes. Then cross them the other way and do the same thing again. I also found some more complex yoga moves that stretched the band more completely like pigeon and cow face (www.yogajournal.com).

The problem is that once you have injured yourself, the stretching may actually aggravate the pain instead of helping it. Often the best solution is to let it heal gradually and then add the stretching exercises in when you are ready to start working out again. Please, don't think that once the problem is gone, you don't have to worry about it anymore. If you don't do the proper stretching exercises, it will recur and you will be frustrated. This is something you have to deal with on a daily basis. Stretching for five to ten minutes a day is a great investment in your health and your continued ability to work out without injury.

Knee Pain

If your pain isn't caused by IT Band issues, you could have a problem with your bike set up. It costs about two hundred dollars to have a professional properly set up your bike. This may sound outrageous when your bike didn't cost two hundred dollars. You may need a new bike, as well. But the bike set up will help you avoid a lot of pain. If your seat is too high, you will feel pain in the front of your knee. If it is too low, you will feel pain in the back. Check this out before you do anything else.

If you know the pain is not a result of poor bike set-up, you may need to see a specialty sports doctor if it continues. Don't just go to your regular family doctor, however. A family doctor doesn't know a lot about sports injuries and may be tempted to tell you to just stop biking or running. A sports doctor is there to help you keep going.

Achilles Heel/Plantar Fasciitis

If you feel pain in your heel or in your foot, especially in the morning when you first take steps, you probably have this problem. The solution is to rest and heal, and then to do proper stretching daily. Lean your foot against the wall at an angle and press on the top of it gently for several minutes each day. Switch and do the other foot. You can also do downward facing dog from yoga (www.yogajournal.com). See a specialty sports doctor if it persists to make sure of a diagnosis. Don't ignore this pain! Never ignore pain. Pain is your body's signal that something is wrong.

If it is Achilles Heel or Plantar Fasciitis, you will need to deal with it on a regular basis. Some people buy a special sock (often called "The Strassburg sock") that stretches the muscles through the night as you sleep. This can be a great temporary solution, but you will need to continue the stretching after you stop wearing the sock. And don't just do stretching before or after you work out. Do stretching separately every day. Flexibility is an important indicator of good health and you should set aside time to do stretching on a daily basis, whether or not you are racing in triathlon. Do it while you are watching TV. Find the time and invest it. Your body will thank you.

Other Pain

Some pains may be alleviated by simply correcting your running stride. If you count how many times your right foot strikes the ground while running for one minute, it should be ninety to one hundred. If it isn't, you need to shorten your stride. Reaching out too far for your stride while running can cause terrible imbalances in the way your body loads weight.

If you are having shoulder pain while swimming, try using a shallower and faster stroke. Also, you can focus on kicking if you need time to heal a shoulder. Shoulder injuries will respond well to RICE therapy.

Again, please do not continue to train and ignore an injury!! The great thing about being a triathlete is that no matter what you have injured, you can probably still find an exercise you can do that will help your training. Work around the pain, not through it.

ABOUT THE AUTHOR

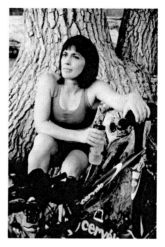

Nationally published Young Adult fiction author Mette Ivie Harrison (*The Princess and the Hound* and *Mira, Mirror*) has been involved in triathlon since 2004, when she won 1st place in her age group at the first triathlon she ever entered. Since 2006, when she finished her first Ironman in 13:02 at Coeur d'Alene, Idaho, she has competed in three other Ironman competitions, six ultramarathons, the longest single day bike race in the United States (LoToJa), and dozens of Olympic and sprint distance races. She is currently nationally ranked by the USAT for her age group and if she doesn't bring home a medal, her children usually know it's because she had a bike crash or was running a fever. Her husband has caught the Ironman bug and has competed in two Ironmans with her. Her four oldest children (ages 12–18) have all competed in either sprint or Olympic distance triathlons or half marathons. She trains them, as well as other family members and friends, writing training plans, and talking them through the hard times.

ABOUT FAMILIUS

Welcome to a place where mothers are celebrated, not compared. Where heart is at the center of our families, and family at the center of our homes. Where boo boos are still kissed, cake beaters are still licked, and mistakes are still okay. Welcome to a place where books—and family—are beautiful. Familius: a book publisher dedicated to helping families be happy.

Familius was founded in 2012 with the intent to align the founders' love of publishing and family with the digital publishing renaissance which occurred simultaneously with the Great Recession. The founders believe that the traditional family is the basic unit of society, and that a society is only as strong as the families that create it.

Familius' mission is to help families be happy. We invite you to participate with us in strengthening your family by being part of the Familius family. Go to www.familius.com to subscribe and receive information about our books, articles, and videos.

Website: www.familius.com
Facebook: www.facebook.com/paterfamilius
Twitter: @familiustalk, @paterfamilius1
Pinterest: www.pinterest.com/familius

CPSIA information can be obtained at www.ICGtesting.com
Printed in the USA
BVOW071418150513

320798BV00001B/4/P